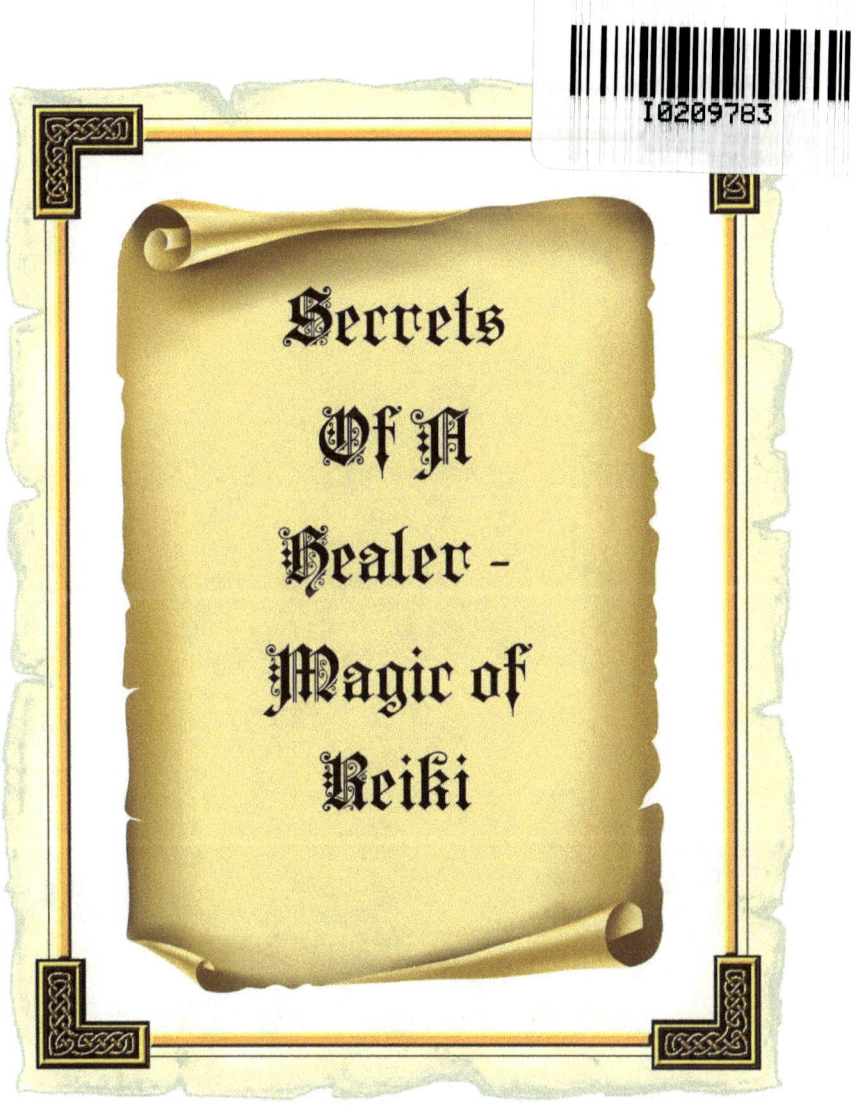

Secrets Of A Healer - Magic of Reiki

Secrets of a Healer

VOL. VIII
MAGIC OF REIKI

Dr. Constance Santego

Maximillian Enterprises
Kelowna, BC

Secrets Of A Healer – Magic of Reiki
Copyright © 2020 by Dr. Constance Santego.

All rights reserved. No part of this publication may be reproduced, distributed, or transmitted in any form or by any means, including photocopying, recording, or other electronic or mechanical methods, without the prior written permission of the publisher, except in the case of brief quotations embodied in critical reviews and certain other noncommercial uses permitted by copyright law. For permission requests, write to the publisher, addressed "Attention: Permissions Coordinator," at the address below.

Copy Editor and Interior Design: Constance Santego
Book Layout: ©2017 BookDesignTemplates.com
Cover Design: Jennifer Louie

Ordering Information:
Quantity sales. Special discounts are available on quantity purchases by corporations, associations, and others. For details, contact the address below.

Trade paperback ISBN: 978-1-7772220-0-0

eBook ISBN 978-1-7772220-1-7

Created and published In Canada. Printed and bound in the United States of America

First Edition
Published by Maximillian Enterprises
Kelowna, BC Canada
www.constancesantego.ca

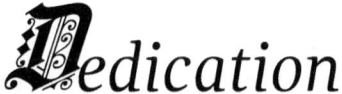

Dedication

To Nefertiti, my first Reiki Instructor, and all other instructors and practitioners that practice this marvelous hands-on-healing technique.

Your hands hold the power to heal.

–Constance Santego

ALSO BY DR. CONSTANCE SANTEGO

FICTION
The Nine Spiritual Gifts Series:

Journey of a Soul – (Vol. 1 Michael)
Language of a Soul – (Vol. 2 Gabriel)
Prophecy of a Soul – (Vol. 3 Bath Kol)
Healing of a Soul – (Vol. 4 Raphael)

NON-FICTION
The Intuitive Life, The Gift of Prophecy, Third Edition

Fairy Tales, Dreams and Reality... Where Are You On Your Path? Second Edition
Your Persona... The Mask You Wear
Angelic Lifestyle, A Vibrant Lifestyle
Angelic Lifestyle 42-Day Energy Cleanse
Archangel Michael's Soul Retrieval Guide

SECRETS OF A HEALER, SERIES:

Magic of Aromatherapy (Vol. I)
Magic of Reflexology (Vol. II)
Magic of The Gifts (Vol. III)
Magic of Muscle Testing (Vol. IV)
Magic of Iridology (Vol. V)
Magic of Massage (Vol. VI)
Magic of Hypnotherapy (Vol. VII)
Magic of Reiki (Vol. VIII)
Magic of Advanced Aromatherapy (Vol. IX)
Magic of Esthetics (Vol. X)

FOR CHILDREN

I am big tonight. I don't need the light!

Contents

Preface xiii
Note to Reader xv
Learning Outcome xvii
PART ONE 1
What is Reiki? 3
    Reiki = Life-Force Energy 4
    Energy 9
    Sensing Energy 15
    Proof of Energy 17
    Benefits of Reiki 18
    Who Can Use Reiki 19
Chakra's 20
    Colors of the Rainbow 22
    Chakra Imbalances 27
    Physical Chakra Imbalances 29
    Emotional & Mental Chakra Imbalances 31
    Spiritual Chakra Imbalances 32
    Quantum Medicine 33
    The Seven Main Chakras 35
    Root Chakra 36
    Sacral Chakra 44
    Solar Plexus Chakra 52
    Heart Chakra 59
    Throat Chakra 66
    Brow Chakra 73
    Crown Chakra 80
PART TWO 87

History of Hands-on-Healing 88
Dr. Usui's Reiki Method 91
Levels of Reiki 96
Lineage 98
How Reiki Energy Works 99
Sensing The Reiki Energy 103
Basics of Level I Reiki 105
Reiki Master in Spirit 108
Reiki Level I Attunement 109
Kidney Breathing & The Hui Yin 110
Water Ritual 111
Raku Kei Affirmation 111
21-Day Cleanse 112

PART THREE 113
Reiki Self-Treatment 114
A Reiki Mantra 117
Reiki Breathing Exercise 118
Reiki Quick Energizer 119
Reiki For Your Electronics 120
Reiki For Your Pets 121
Reiki For Your Plants 122
Reiki For Sleep 123
Aromatherapy For Chakras 124
Chakra Stone Technique 125
Crystal Chakra Release 128
Muscle Testing Chakra *for* Meditation 129
Negative Energy & Chakra Clearing Meditation 130
Pendulum Chakra Release 135
Sound Essence Chakra Balancers 136

  Tuning Forks Chakra Balance 138
  BONUS - Healing Pool 140
Charts 143
  Energy 144
  Feelings 145
  Meridians 146
  Musical Notes 147
  Organs & Glands 148
  Senses 149
Bibliography 151
Message From The Author 164

Preface

The Miracle of Reiki

In 1999, Reiki was one of the first modalities taught in my new school. I did not know what Reiki was until Nefertiti came and offered Level I & II in my school. It was an amazing weekend course that altered my life forever.

You must understand that back then, all this "stuff" was woo, hocus pocus stuff. And to most people, Reiki was still believed to be the Devil's work.

It is bizarre that people say something is of the Devil just because they do not understand what they cannot see, feel, hear, or know to be true or beneficial. I find that humanity is quite a fickle society. When I grew up, marijuana was bad, and now it is medicinal.

I am so happy and grateful that Reiki is now one of those things society has changed its mind upon!

Note to Reader

Reiki is not intended to replace traditional medical techniques. Persons with physical, mental, emotional, and spiritual problems should seek the service of a professional psychologist or Doctor.

Your Doctor still plays a vital role in your health care. For example, if I break my leg, I will need a Doctor, all the nurses, and staff that work in the Hospital.

Integrated Medicine focuses on the fact that **we play** a significant role in caring for our health. What we put into our bodies, how hard we work our bodies, the stress level we allow into our everyday life, and the positive or negative energy we attract around us all play a role in our wellbeing.

Reiki is an excellent technique for relaxation, stress relief, clearing the mind, improving self-awareness, self-empowerment, and possibly a miracle. However, you are ALWAYS in control of your health, and Reiki has no power to heal you on its own. Only you can do that.

Shift happens…Create magic!

Learning Outcome

When you have completed this book, studied the concepts and techniques, and participated in the online Reiki Level I attunement, you will be able to perform the self-healing techniques of Reiki (to help reduce stress, relax sore and achy muscles, and empower your body, mind, and soul).

- What is Reiki,
- Energy Healing,
- Hands-on-Healing techniques,
- And many other techniques to balance your Chakras and Tsubus.

PART ONE

2 DR. CONSTANCE SANTEGO

What is Reiki?

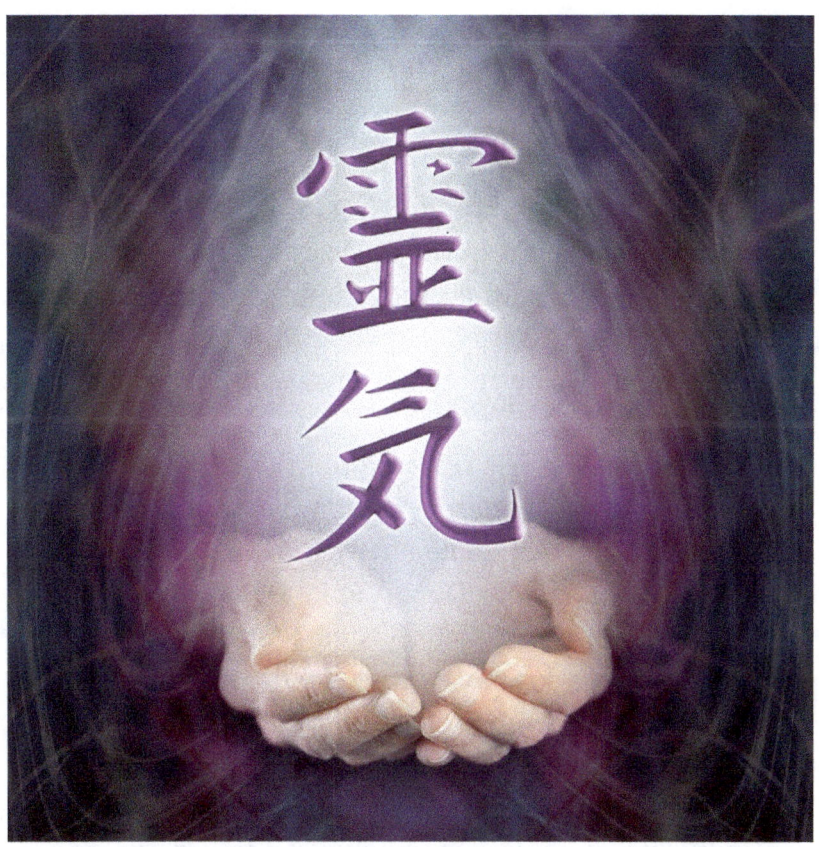

Reiki is a hands-on-healing energy technique used on the body's chakras and tsubus (meridian points).

Reiki = Life-Force Energy

Reiki is one of the most ancient healing methods known to mankind, used as an alternative therapy for treating physical, emotional, mental, and spiritual dis-ease.

Reiki is the Japanese word for 'Universal Life-force Energy.' The definition of 'Rei' is a universal, mysterious power, transcendental spirit. 'Ki' is described as the vital life-force energy. Together they could mean 'Spirit Energy' or 'Power Energy.' However, the essence is more that of 'Universal Life-force Energy – All-Encompassing.'

The tradition of Reiki is referred to in the 3500-year-old writings in Sanskrit, where writing was used as a means of communication and dialogue by the Hindu Celestial Gods and was termed as Deva-Vani ('Deva' Gods - 'Vani' language) as it was believed to have been generated by the God Brahma who passed it to the Rishis (sages) living in celestial bodies, who then communicated the same to their earthly disciples from where it spread on earth. Today it is used by the Indo-Aryans (the ancient language in Hinduism), and it is also widely used in Jainism, Buddhism, and Sikhism.

Reiki is not a religion or belief system – it holds no doctrine. It is a healing modality that combines the power of God's life-force healing energy and your body's Chakra system.

Where does this universal life-force energy come from?

In science, the specific energy used in Reiki falls under the electromagnetic field category. This is because Reiki energy has a vibration, frequency, and wavelength of energy, just like many things on Earth.

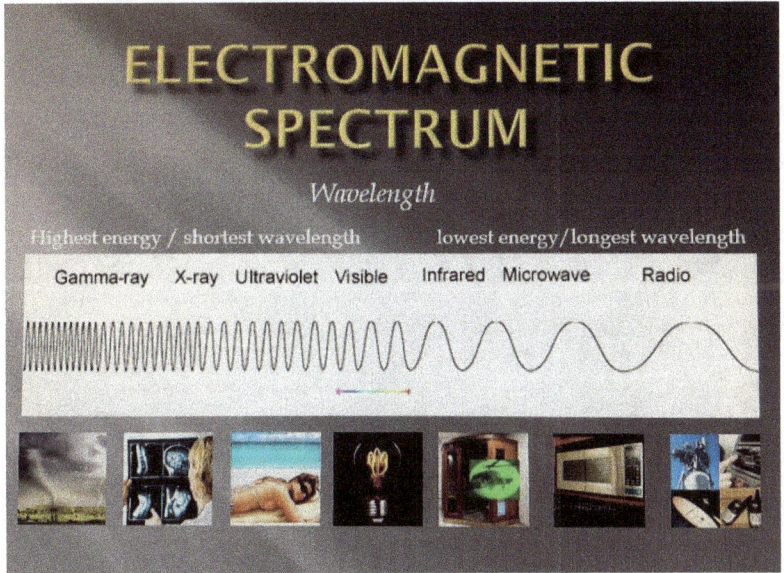

I am getting to the good stuff; bear with me.

In 1665, Francesco Maria Grimaldi, an Italian Jesuit priest, conducted a simple experiment of light entering a dark room through a small slit and projecting onto a white screen. Not only was the beam of light illuminating the screen larger than expected, it was no longer white but became two or three rays of different colors.

In 1666, Isaac Newton passed sunlight through a prism, split the light beam into different colors, and was the first to understand that white light consists of a mix of light rays, each with a different color.

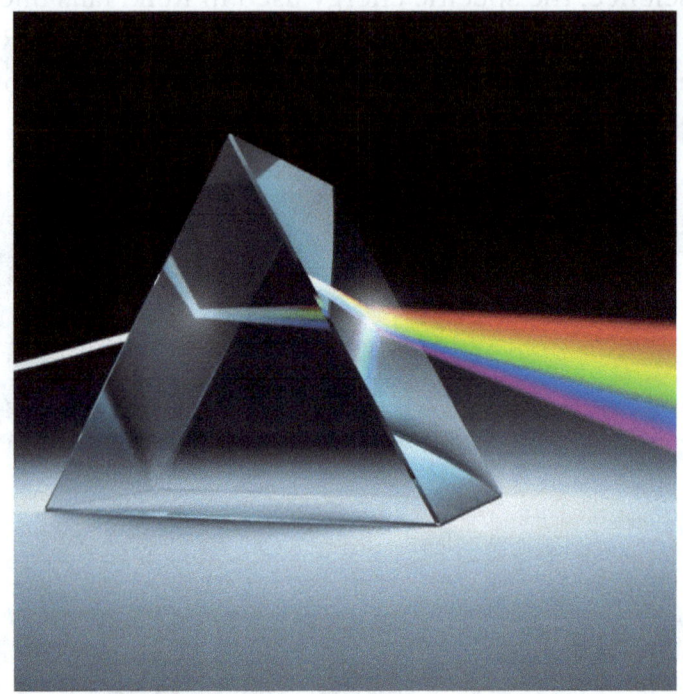

The white light's ray breaks into the seven primary colors of a rainbow:

Color	Tera Hertz
1. Red	435 - 495
2. Orange	495 - 515
3. Yellow	515 - 535
4. Green	535 - 630
5. Blue	630 - 660
6. Indigo	660 - 680
7. Violet	680 - 740

Here is why scientific information matters. In Reiki, this colored life-force energy emanates from the Heavens (God, Spirit, creator, the universe, or any other name you call God) to not only feed and grow healthy plants, but a person performing Reiki uses this specific group of rays to feed, grow, and heal ourselves, others, and the planet.

Each ray of colored energy has a unique healing frequency.

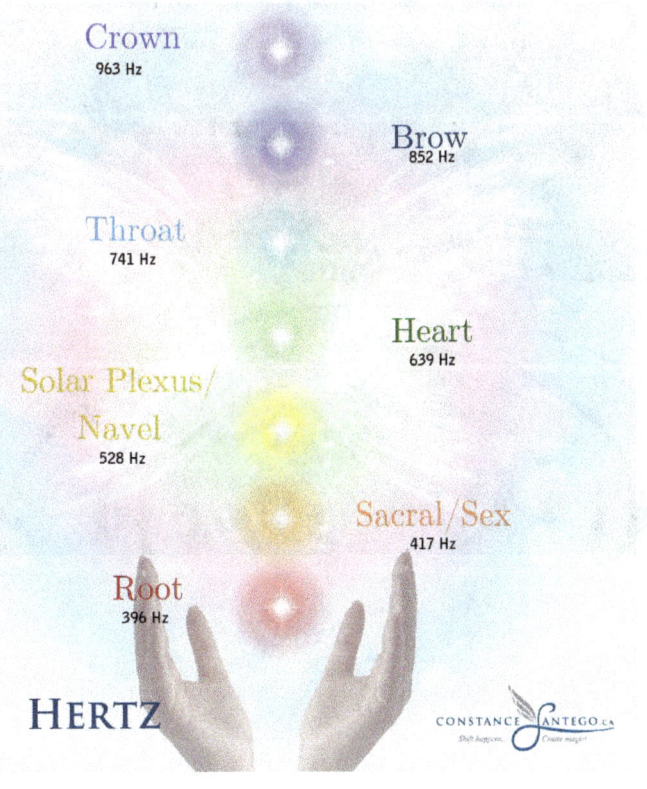

HERTZ

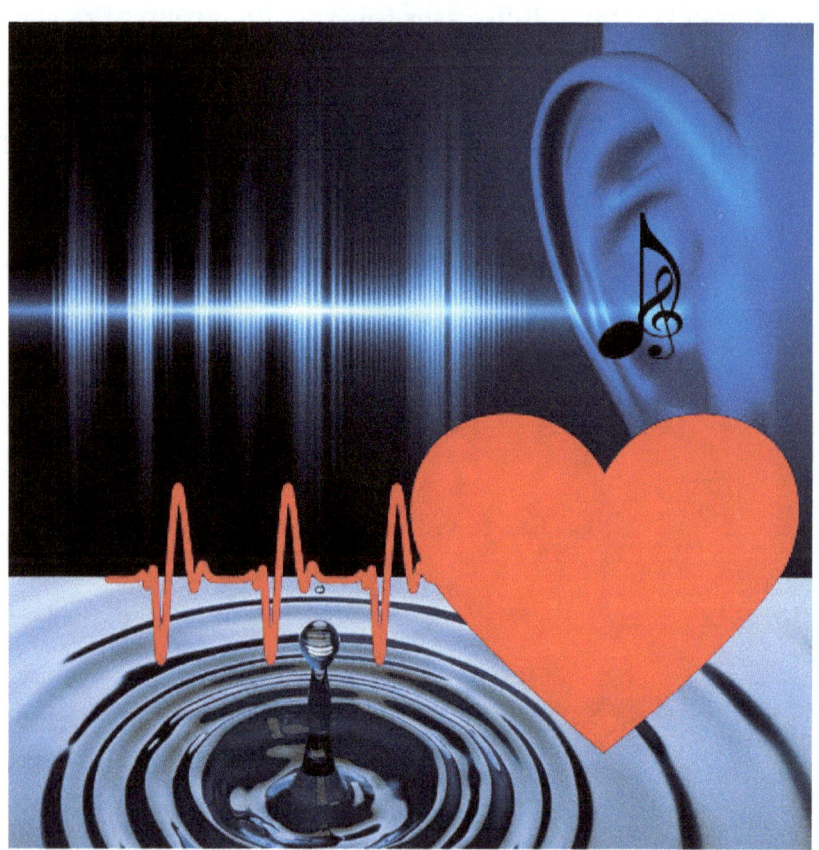

Energy

Energy healing is not new and is becoming increasingly accepted in the modern medical world.

Many hospitals accept Reiki practitioners to perform energy healing sessions on their Cancer patients.

Vibrational healing is based on the electromagnetic field of the human body. All atoms in your body must have equal protons and negative electrons orbiting a neutron to be stable and healthy.

Every cell in your body is made up of elements, which make up atoms, which make up molecules in your body (heart cells, muscles, bones, nerves, liver, etc.). The elements creating the different atoms and molecules vibrate at different hertz frequencies.

Read this next part carefully!!! When a person suffers from a health condition or dis-ease (stress, sickness, trauma, or has been contaminated), the exact number of negative electrons circling the atom are displaced, creating an imbalance of energy around the atom. Suppose available negative ions are not near the unstable atom to replenish it. In that case, the atom will move through your body, tearing it up and looking for another negative ion to become stable again. This action damages your body and creates dis-ease, premature aging, and free radical damage. You may even notice the signs of free radical damage being done by liver spots or age spots appearing on your hands and arms. Or you can be tested with a biofeedback machine.

The application of using frequencies to heal the body was originally suggested by the American inventor **Nikola Tesla** (1856 – 1943), who pioneered electrical technology. And back in the late 1920s, **Dr. Royal R. Rife** found that specific frequencies could prevent disease development and that other frequencies would destroy disease. He invented and built the Rife machine – one of the first frequency generators. Using his invention, he found that substances with a higher frequency would destroy the disease of a lower frequency. Unfortunately for the millions of people with Cancer, and like Nikola Tesla's fate, Dr. Rife's office was broken into, all his paperwork and research were stolen, and the burglars destroyed his Rife machine.

More recently, **Bruce Tainio of Tainio Technology**, an independent division of Eastern State University in Cheney, Washington, 1992 built the first frequency monitor in the world. He also agrees that every disease has a frequency. He agreed with Tesla's and Rife's findings that the hertz frequency of disease in the body is lower than the normal healthy body's 62-72' hertz.

Disease
- Colds and Flu start at: 57-60 MHz
- Disease starts at: 58 MHz
- Candida overgrowth starts at: 55 MHz
- Receptive to Epstein Barr at: 52 MHz
- Receptive to Cancer at: 42 MHz
- Death begins at: 25 MHz

Healthy
- Genius Brain Frequency 80-82 MHz
- Brain Frequency Range 72-90 MHz
- Normal Brain Frequency 72 MHz
- Human Body 62-78 MHz
- Human Body: from Neck up 72-78 MHz
- Human Body: from Neck down 60-68 MHz
- Thyroid and Parathyroid glands are 62-68 MHz
- Thymus Gland is 65-68 MHz
- Heart is 67-70 MHz
- Lungs are 58-65 MHz
- Liver is 55-60 MHz
- Pancreas is 60-80 MHz

The study of frequencies raises an important question concerning the frequencies of substances we eat, breathe, and absorb—many pollutants lower healthy frequencies.
- Processed/canned food has a frequency of zero,
- Fresh produce has up to 15 Hz,
- Dried herbs from 12 to 22 Hz,
- Fresh herbs from 20 to 27 Hz.

The exciting part is that these displaced electrons are what scientists have proven to make up your vital or auric field, your aura. These electrons create your auric field and vibrate at different hertz frequencies, depending on your state of mind and health.

Dr. Valerie Virginia Hunt, Ed. D (July 22, 1916 – February 24, 2014) was a scientist, author, and former professor of Physiological Science at the University of California, Los Angeles. She is best known for her pioneering research in the field of **bioenergy.**

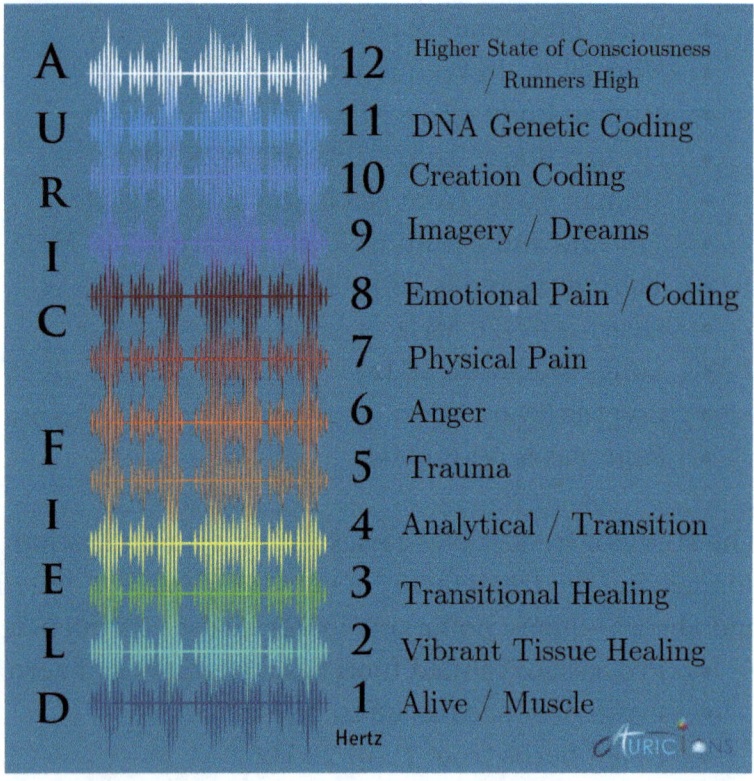

One of her videos talks about the vital or auric field's color (different from *a Chakra color)*.
- 1200 hertz is a higher state of consciousness
- 900 - 1200 hertz - high blue (indigo) and violet
- 700-800 hertz - red and pain (genetic coding/DNA)
- 600 hertz - orange and anger
- 400 hertz - yellow and needed for a transition
- 300 hertz - green
- 100 hertz - blue and the vibration of a person's muscle

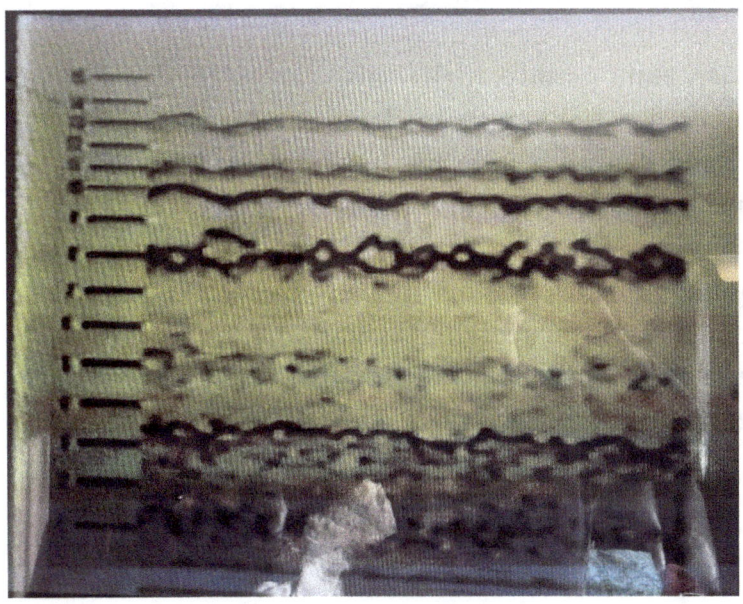

To heal, Dr. Hunt says a subtle frequency shift needs to happen (as in the shift that will occur during a massage, acupressure, or laying on of hands session).

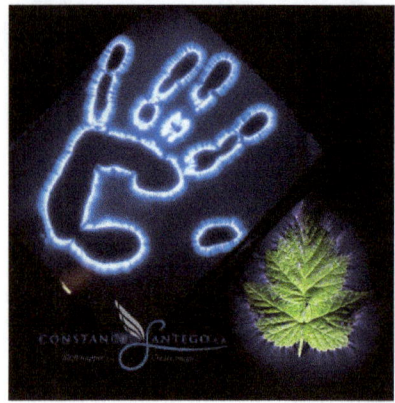

You probably already have heard about **Kirlian photography**. It is a collection of photographic techniques used to capture the phenomenon of electrical corona discharges, also known as the auric field of an object. The color of the glow around the object can change depending on the vibrational frequency or the hertz the item vibrates at.

As in Dr. Hunt's study, Kirlian also agreed that an aura or human energy field emanates from the surface of an object and that each color has been proven to have a different hertz frequency.

My point is that there is a science to back up the healing power achieved through hertz manipulation from a healer's hands-on-healing session. And even though not all people can see, feel, know, or hear the healing being done, Reiki is a scientifically proven modality.

Sensing Energy

THOUGHT ENERGY

The following couple of exercises will help you notice energy.

Exercise #1

1. Walk around the room like you usually do.
2. *Notice how you feel.*
3. Stop and take a breath.
4. Now have your intent or thought change to imagine while you are walking this time, your feet have cords that grow out of them like tree roots, and they grow to the center of the earth.
5. Now walk and notice what you sense this time. Any difference? *Notice how you feel.*
6. Stop again and take a breath.
7. Now have your intent change to imagining you are walking as if you are as light as a feather, with no weight.
8. Again, walk around and notice what you sense this time. Any difference? *Notice how you feel.*
9. Once you have tried all three, take a breath, let go of the experience, and return to your original self or how you want to be.

Exercise #2

1. With a partner, stand facing each other. Have your partner stand normal.
2. Test their energy. Lightly with your hand, move the other person's shoulder. Push them lightly backward.
3. Now have them take a breath and imagine that their feet have cords that go out of them like tree roots that tie to the earth's center.
4. Now lightly with your hand, move them to their shoulder. Push them backward again.
5. *Notice any difference?*
6. Next, have them breathe and imagine they are as light as a feather.
7. Then lightly with your hand, move them to their shoulder. Lightly push them backward again. (be careful not to push them over where they fall, LIGHTLY).
8. *Notice any difference?*

If you do not notice any difference, try a few different people. The purpose of the exercises is to show you what you think can change your energy field. Yes, even gravitational.

Interesting! What we think is what we create. As I say, "Be careful what you think. You might just get it."

Proof of Energy

There are many toys that prove that YOU, all by yourself, can conduct energy. This 'Energy Stick' is fun to show my students how Reiki energy works. You can buy these at Walmart, Toys 'R' US, or online.

- You can make it light up and play a song by holding one hand at each end and touching the metal.
- I have done this with fourteen students holding hands. Two of us are holding one end each.
  - The really cool part is when someone breaks contact with the link, and the toy instantly turns off.
  - Then when they touch hands again, it instantly plays again.
  - It only works, though, if you are touching skin to skin. It doesn't work through clothing.

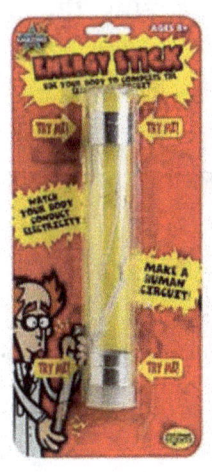

Exercise #3

*You can see a demo on my Constance Santego YouTube Channel, "Proof of Energy," Experiment #1

Benefits of Reiki

Reiki can and will benefit your
Body, Mind & Soul!

As I said earlier, the benefits of Reiki are becoming well-known in Hospitals and Cancer clinics. Many stories are being told of mystical healings and peace of mind coming from these sessions.

Out of all the modalities I know how to do, Reiki has the most outstanding results, miracles, some might say! I have witnessed the healing gift of Spirit through Reiki. Many, many times, I have witnessed pain disappearing forever, hearing coming back, eyesight improving, the diagnosed tumor of breast Cancer turning into goo, and then days later disappearing.

One never knows what is going to happen in a Reiki session. It is not up to me to decide what is going to happen. Spirit decides. God, your Angels, and Guides are the ones who deliver this life-force healing energy. All I can do is follow my instincts regarding where to place my hands.

Who Can Use Reiki

We are all born with the ability or gift to use the universal life-force healing energy. When you hurt yourself, what is your first reaction (other than cursing), putting your hand on the area that is in pain? This action helps to lessen the pain or to relieve it altogether.

The healing energy used in Reiki is gentle yet immensely powerful. It heals by balancing and harmonizing your body, mind, or soul's vibration or frequency. The universal life-force energy coming to your hands will shift and balance the person's vital field (aura), affecting each Chakra.

Anybody can learn how to use Reiki. However, I would suggest a mature person understand two things. First, how to focus their intention of bringing this healing energy into their body and out of their hands, and second, they can do this without giving away their energy. Yes, you can give away your power! But, if you do not bring in the extra life-force energy into your body, you will not have enough to stay healthy or let alone heal someone.

You will know if you have given away your energy or taken on their energy because you will feel weak, tired, or even sick after a session. Reiki is to be used as a one-way channel. NEVER take the other person's energy!!! A way to help you achieve this is not to touch the other person but to hover over them.

Chakra's

Chakra is a Sanskrit word used by Hindus, meaning 'wheel of light.' Most traditions refer to seven major Chakras within the body.

Clairvoyants (French for clear vision), these people are born with the gift of sight. They can perceive Chakras and describe them as circular spirals of energy, which differ in size and vibrate at different frequencies.

Chakras serve as gateways, portals, or transformers to collect and absorb the flow of assimilated energy into our physical bodies. Our material bodies could not exist without them.

In the Eastern Medicine practices of Chinese Medicine and Aura Vedic Medicine, it is believed that Chakras connect the life-force energy from the cosmos to the human body through the meridian system. Meridians are channels through which life-force energy runs to energize and balance each organ in the body.

Our Chakras are funnel-shaped spinning energy vortexes of multicolored light. Each Chakra in the body attracts, emanates, and transforms this light energy into a specific color frequency.

Imagine a Chakra is a whirlwind, where cosmic life-force energy flows into and out of in the middle of this whirlwind.

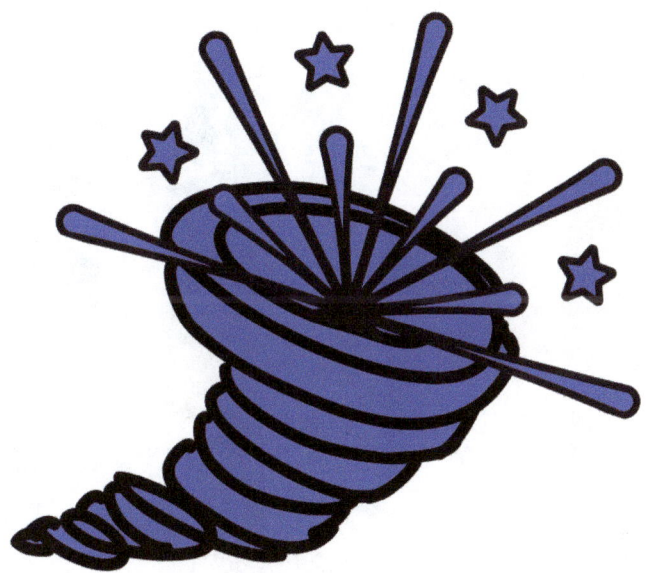

Chakras act as pressure valves for this subtle life-force energy system.

Colors of the Rainbow

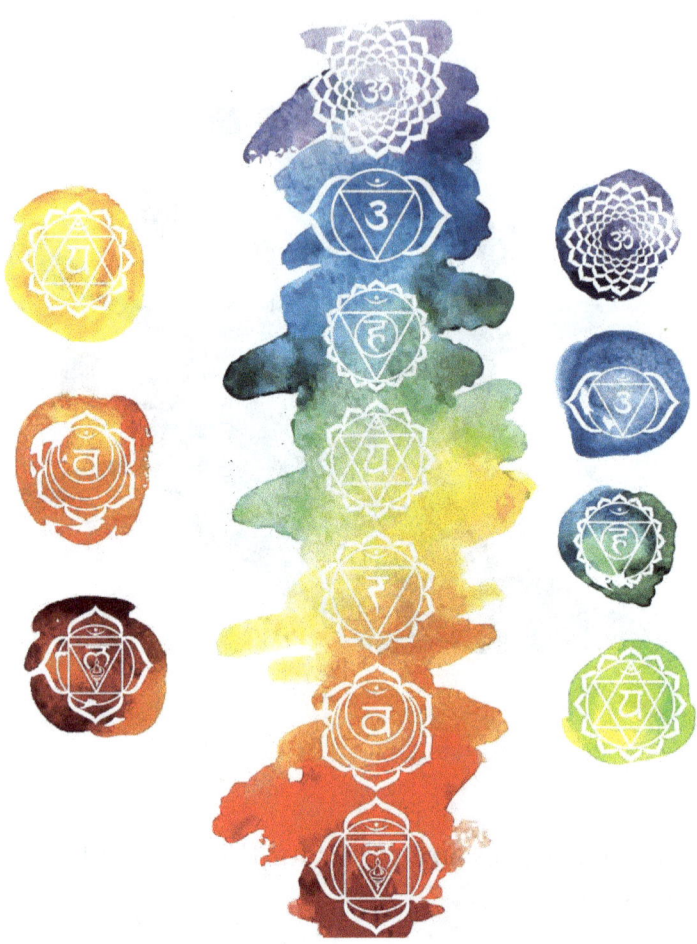

Color Wheel – Complementary Colors

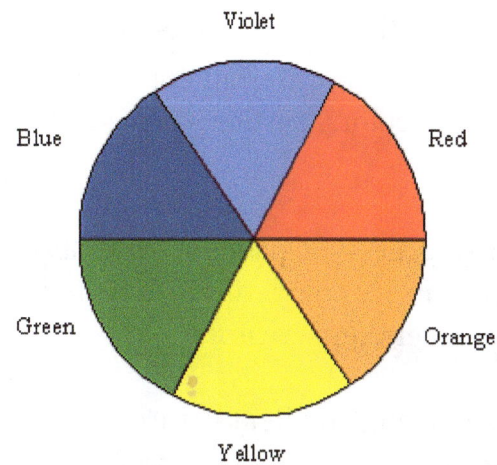

Colors of the Rainbow and Chakras

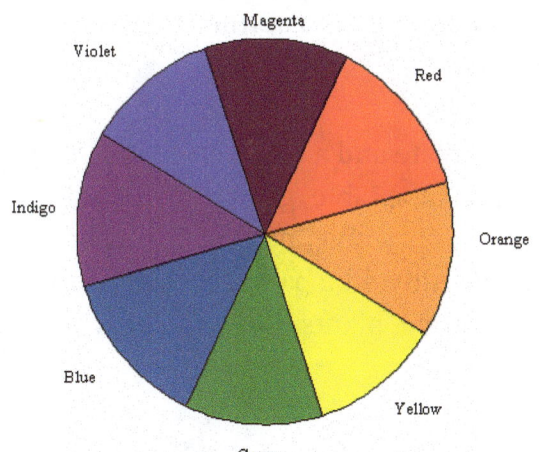

*The seven main Chakras; red, orange, yellow, green, blue, indigo, and violet (new to the rainbow is magenta. Connecting red and violet is magenta).

Meanings of the Chakra Colors

There are seven layers of the Auric body. As you learn each of them, notice they can be different colors. So, if you and a friend see other colors, ensure which auric field you are viewing.

Red: energizing, vitalizing, heating, passion, material generosity, vigor, force, highly competitive, outgoing, assertive, initiators, pioneers, and creators.

Orange: enthusiastic, buoyant, ebullient nature, open-minded, emotional, sensuous, joyful, spontaneity, cheerfulness, talkative, outgoing, sociable, warm-hearted, generally excitable with a happy disposition.

Yellow: supersensitive people, highly nervous, optimistic, intelligent, very capable in business, too generous, sense of reason, logic, and assessment, grasp things quickly, controlling, and dominating.

Green: need to communicate and a lot of affection, very independent, thoughtful, adaptable, growth-oriented, neither dominating nor submissive, neither extrovert nor introvert, balanced, neat, tidy, like parks, coasts, open spaces, wood, clay and stone, plants, flowers, self-control, sympathy, and sharing.

Blue: a sense of well-being, soft, gentle, peaceful by nature, passive, introverted, value truth, honesty, trustworthy, reliable, faithful, too self-absorbed, the order in life and structure, artistic, creative, loyal, sincere, fall in love 100%, harmonious, imaginative, serene, tactful, and daydream.

Indigo: alive, energetic, mystic, psychic, and intuitive.

Violet: spiritual consciousness, awareness, and healers.

Magenta: kindness, gentleness, consideration, affection, warmth, compassion, love, maturity, deep understanding of life, encouraging others to reach their full potential, cooperative, friendly, genuine, counseling, nursing, social work, unconditional love, and affection.

Other Important Colors:

Black: power, authority, knowledge, prestige, negative thoughts, discord, hate, emotional disturbance, death, grief, patience, and can attract negative spirits.

Brown: great energy, logic, analysis, self-starters, moneymakers, very impatient, earthy, stable, grounded, inner confidence, and self-assuredness, dedicated, committed to their family, work, and friends, practical, materialistic, organized, steadfast, "no-nonsense."

Grey: a balance between white and black, maturity, fear, depression, reflecting caution, dull and somber.

Pink: quiet, refined, modest, beautiful, gifted, great devotion, and much self-sacrifice.

Purple: extremely sensitive, non-judgmental, seekers, Unity (love, intellect, and faith).

Silver: enjoy peace, serenity, sedative, lovers of convention, and formality.

Turquoise: unfulfilled ambitions, spiritually protected, sparkling youthfulness, imagination, an attitude of "take it in stride," decisions are made quickly, clarity, insight, need to be more grounded.

White: spiritually elevated, motivated, with an air of cleanliness, purity, innocence, and detachment. It reflects all colors.

Chakra Imbalances

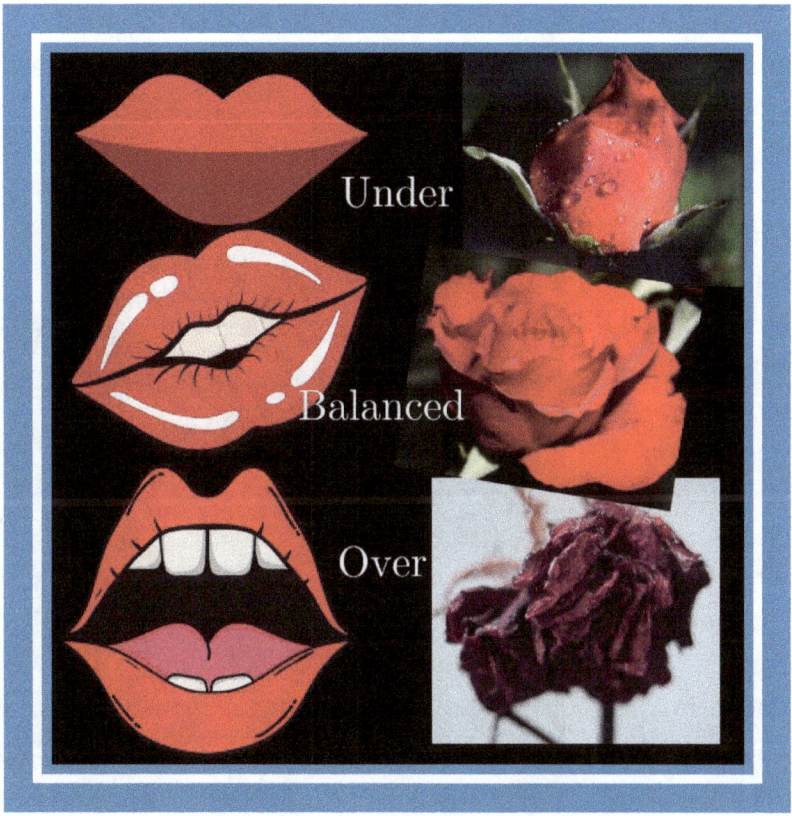

Your Chakras react to every influence coming from your external world. These influences shift your internal body, mind, or soul, which can close or open the Chakras accordingly.

When the body is in dis-ease (disease), it is believed that one or more Chakras' energy flow is blocked, depleted, or an excess of energy enters the meridian channel.

When out of balance, our bodies will be in a flux of sympathetic (fight & flight) or parasympathetic (rest & repair) states. This state of being can lead to an imbalance and disharmony on your physical, mental, emotional, and spiritual levels.

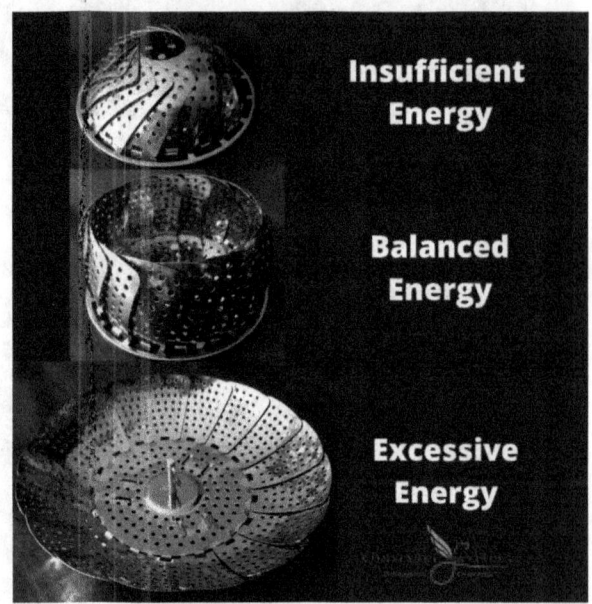

A Closed Chakra (as in the strainer being closed) can cause a blockage, imbalance, or build-up of energy, and when it reaches a certain saturation within each of us, it causes crystallization (pain). Insufficient or excessive energy harms our body, mind, and soul.

Any Chakra Can Be:

- Balanced—in Homeostasis
- Under—Closed or Depleted
- Overflowing—in Excess

Physical Chakra Imbalances

The easiest to tell is when one of your physical Chakras is out of balance.

Chakras that affect your Physical Body
- Root (Base),
- Sacral (Spleen, Sexx),
- Solar Plexus (Navel)

Examples of physical imbalance:
➢ Shoulder pain often occurs when a person feels they are carrying a heavy load of responsibilities.
➢ Ankle pain is associated with flexibility in thought and or action.
➢ Lower back stress is often associated with stress over financial worries.
➢ Gall bladder problems are associated with anger or hurt.

Quantum Medicine also calls the Physical Body the Physical Body.

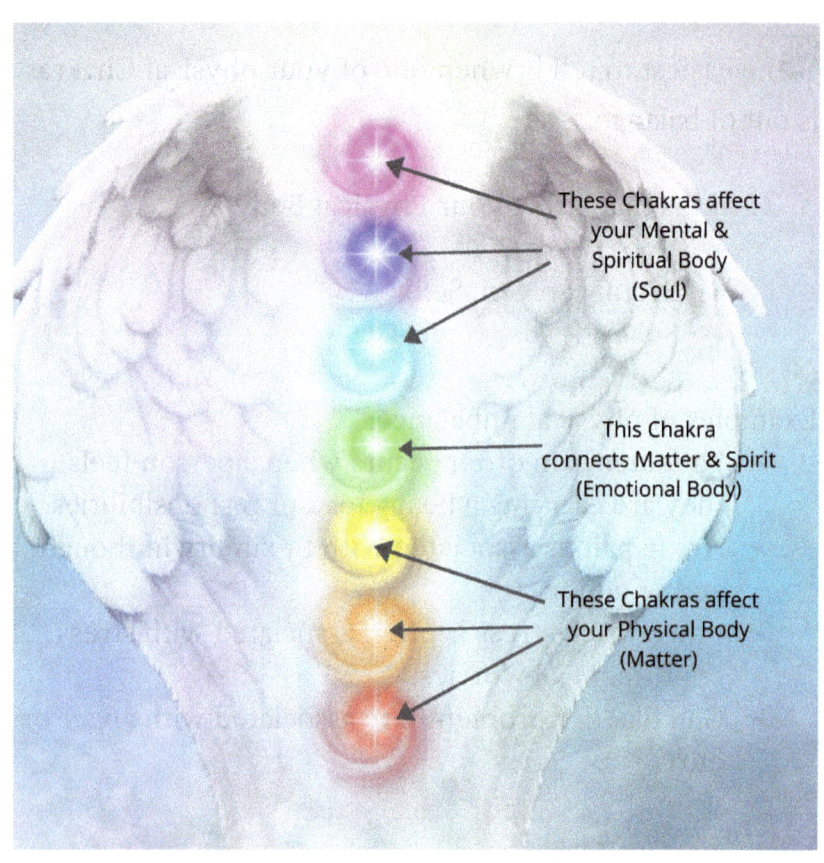

Emotional & Mental Chakra Imbalances

We are emotional beings.

Most people can quickly notice body pain, and they usually go to a Doctor and get a physical problem fixed. BUT what about when it is created because of your emotions? Understanding how emotional difficulties can create disease in the body is based on a broad knowledge of how the Chakras affect your wellbeing.

Chakras that affect your Emotional Body
- Heart
- Throat

Examples of blockages or build-ups:
- Heart pain can mean relationship problems or worry about everyone and everything.
- Memories of past traumas
- Habits and Patterns.
- Freedom of expression

A marvelous reference for emotional causes of dis-ease is Louise Hay's book, 'How to Heal Your Body.'

*Quantum Medicine calls the Emotional Body, Vital Body.

Spiritual Chakra Imbalances

What we think creates our reality, and what we believe affects our thoughts.

Eastern Medicine has a backward concept to our Western beliefs. Here, we believe if we hurt ourselves, it is a physical reason, but Eastern belief is that it is a Spiritual reason.

Chakras that affect your Mental & Spiritual Body
- Brow (Third Eye)
- Crown

Examples of blockages or build-ups:
- Subconscious programming and Beliefs
- Karma from past lifetimes.
- Life Purpose
- Life Lessons.

*Quantum Medicine calls the Spiritual Body, the Bliss Body, and the Mental Body has a Supramental aspect.

Quantum Medicine

Quantum Medicine follows the same belief that Eastern Medicine does.

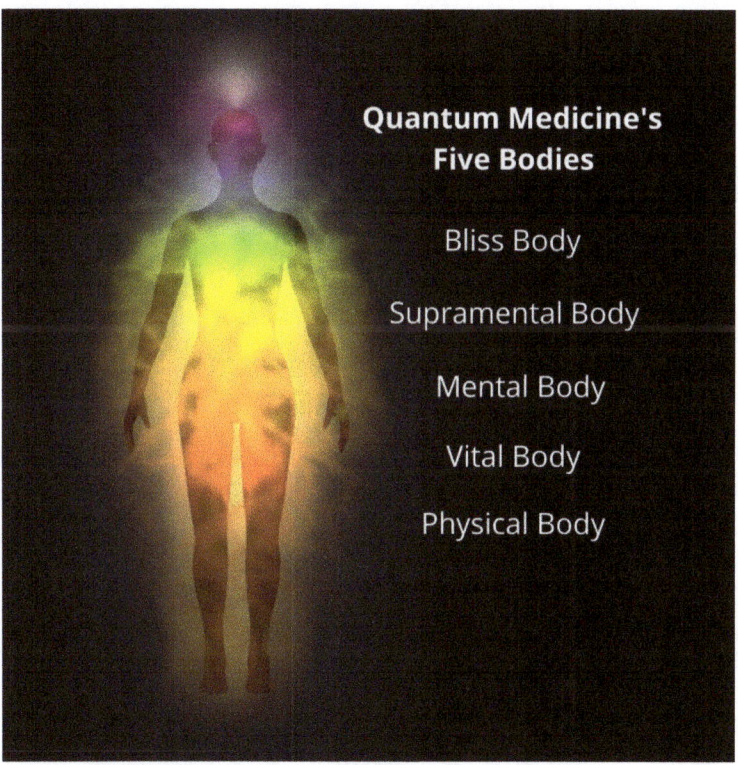

That illness can be the key to understanding and healing the emotional blockages in the body. A healer can simply "purify" the Chakras and balance them so that the body, Mind, and soul's energy flows smoothly.

Bliss Body – God Consciousness
Balancing Techniques
- Belief

Supramental Body – Godly Archetypes
Balancing Techniques
- Tachyon Technologies
- Prayer
- Reiki

Mental Body – Meaning to Life
Balancing Techniques
- Meditation
- Hypnotherapy
- Neuro-Linguistic Programming
- Flower or Bach Remedies

Vital Body – Morphogenetic Field (Aura)
Balancing Techniques
- Chakra
- Color
- Crystals
- Sound

Physical Body – Manifestation
Balancing Techniques
- Negative Ions
- Tuning Forks
- Herbs
- Vitamins
- Medicine
- Biofeedback

The Seven Main Chakras

Reiki uses the body's Chakra system by breaking the energy blockages or excess and then balancing the Body, Mind, and Soul.

1. Root (Base) Chakra
2. Sacral (Spleen, Sexx) Chakra
3. Solar Plexus (Navel) Chakra
4. Heart Chakra
5. Throat Chakra
6. Brow (Third Eye) Chakra
7. Crown Chakra

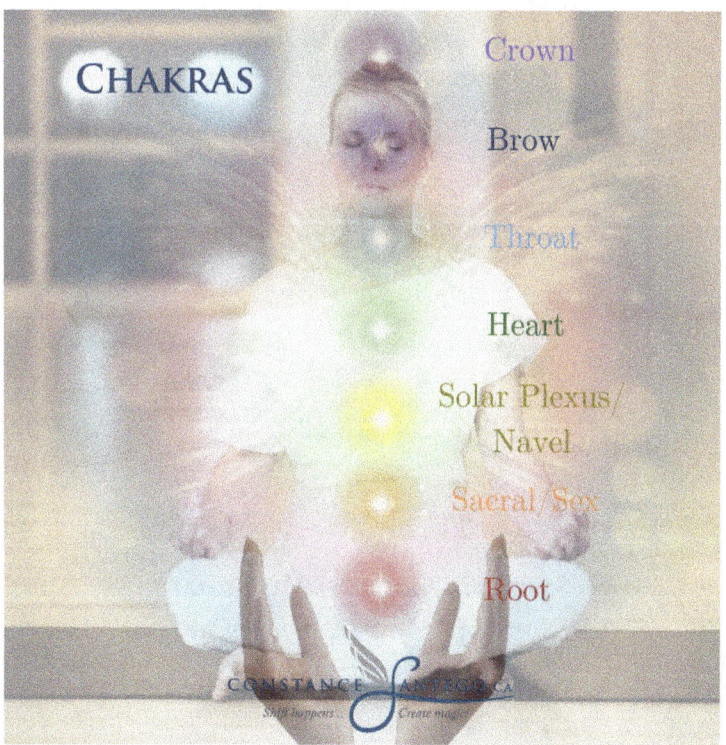

Root Chakra

Also Known As - Base Chakra

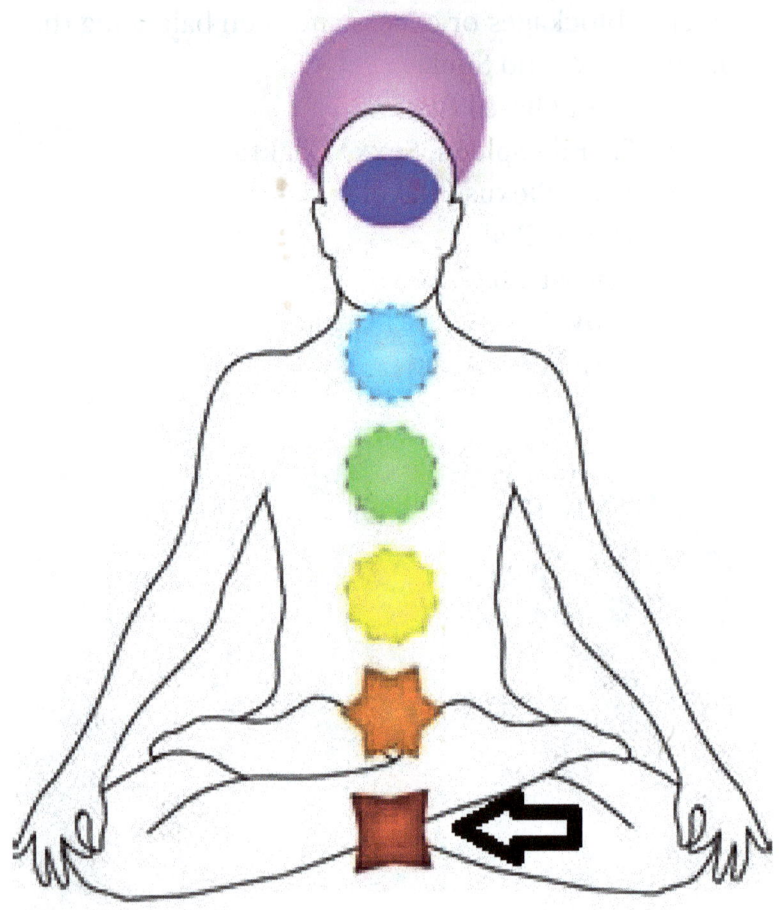

Sanskrit Name Is: Muladhara
The Sanskrit name translates to 'root.'

Root Chakra Symbol:

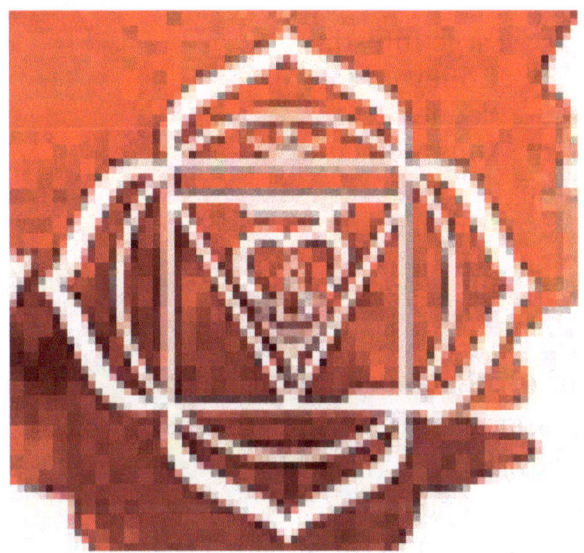

Color in the Rainbow: Red

Hertz Frequency: 396 Hz

Location: 1st of the 7 Chakras is:
- The base of the spine (between anus and genitals).
- It opens downward

Fundamental Meaning:
Vitality, Courage & Self Confidence
- Dominate Feelings - Rootedness & Survival
- Our Personal Energy Source
- All About You and Your Basic Needs

It is associated with our connection to the earth, survival, health, abundance, family, passion, and moving forward in life.

Organs & Glands Controlled by the Root Chakra:

- Organs,
    - Large Intestine
    - Kidney (right)
    - Bladder
    - Anus & Rectum
- Gland
    - Adrenals

Quantum Medicine: Physical Body

Symptoms of a Balanced Root Chakra:
Vibrating Good Health & Homeostasis
- Comfortable in the body
- Well Grounded
- Sense of trust in the world
- Vitality & Health
- Sense of safety and security
- Stability
- Prosperity, Abundance & Wealth

Symptoms of PHYSICAL Imbalances of an Under or Over-Balanced Root Chakra
Dis-ease:
- Retain Water
- Sore Back
- Dry Skin and Hair
- Constipated/Diarrhea
- Burping/Gas
- Poor Circulation
- Constipation.
- Diarrhea.
- Piles

- Colitis
- Crohn's disease
- Cold fingers and toes
- Frequency of urination
- Hypertension (high blood pressure)
- Kidney stones
- Impotence
- Problems with hips, legs, and feet

Symptoms of EMOTIONAL & MENTAL Imbalances of an Under or Over-Balanced Root Chakra Dis-ease:
- Fear
- Trust Issues
- Issues with parents
- Abuse as a child
- Self-confidence Issues
- Apprehension, temper, lack of balance, suppression, and lack of confidence.
- Anger
- Frustration
- Depression

If the root (base) Chakra becomes unbalanced, you may feel "stuck" and cannot move forward in life. You may feel ungrounded, with a depleting sense of self. An imbalanced Root Chakra can cause great insecurity, survival problems such as money or food irritability, and obsession with materialistic aspects.

Symptoms of SPIRITUAL Imbalances of an Under or Over-Balanced Root Chakra
Dis-ease:
- Not able to receive abundance from your God's source

How to Balance the Root Chakra – Body, Mind & Soul

- **Affirmations:**
    - I am perfect just the way I am
    - I am stable and secure
    - I trust my body's wisdom
    - I nurture my body
    - I take full responsibility for my life
- **Aromatherapy:** Cedar, Clove, Pepper, Vetiver
- **Color:** Red. Immerse yourself in red-red clothes, red foods, red oils, red herbs, red gemstones, red lights, red candles, red flowers, and drinking water out of red glasses (see the color, wear the color, draw with the color, think the color, taste the color, smell the color, and hear the color)
- **Communication:** 100% receiving
- **Crystals:** Ruby, Garnet, Red Jasper, Hawk-Eye, Smoky Quartz
- **Hertz:** 256 Hz, Tuning Forks, Biofeedback
- **Incense:** Patchouli, Vetiver, Cedarwood, Myrrh, Sandalwood
- **Meditation:**
    - **Red Candle:** Represent passion and energy.

IDEAS

1) Light a red candle and stare at the flame. Let your mind go for 2 – 5 minutes.

2) Go to my Constance Santego YouTube Channel to watch and listen to the Root Chakra Meditation.
3) Have someone read you this meditation. Find a comfortable place to sit or lie down.

Root Chakra Meditation:

Slowly breathe deeply through your nose.
Let all outside noises disappear... release the tension of the muscles in your feet... breathe in and out... relaxing... relaxing your calves, knees, and thighs... breathe in and out... relaxing even more... letting go of all the tension in your legs... breathing in and out... slowly...

As you relax more and more, you start to feel yourself sinking deeper into whatever you are sitting or lying on... Feeling safe and secure... Now visualize yourself somewhere in the world... in perfect surroundings... whether inside or by water, a meadow, or in the mountains... feeling safe and secure...

Look around and see which angel or guide greets you in this serene place. Acknowledge each one. Feel their love radiate as a reddish glow penetrates every cell of your being... filling you with security, health, and abundance... Imagine seeing your angel or guide looking lovingly down at you. Sense their smile as a kiss of sunshine from Heaven... healing you from the inside out... Know that they will never let you down. They are a part of you and will always protect you...

Approach your angel or guide with a hug, kiss, or high-five... Enjoy the sensation... Feel the love and warmth... Take as much time as you need to get to know one another...

Feel the trust and bond between the two of you... They tell you they have a specific gift to enhance this Chakra for you... Allow your angel or guide to give it to you...

Examine it... feel it, smell it, admire the color and shape... If it is appropriate, even taste it...

Thank your angel or guide and tell them you will always treasure your gift...

It is yours to keep and recall it whenever you feel fear or anger... As you hold your gift, feel the love channeled into your Root Chakra... Focus on the smooth motion of the Chakra rotating in a clockwise or counterclockwise direction... Feel the warm red glow that fills the base of your spine... flowing down your legs, calves, and into your feet... this red energy flows through you into the ground and the earth... Grounding you... Enjoy the wonderful sensation of being blessed by your angels and guides before bringing your attention back to your everyday surroundings...

Take a deep breath and thank your angel or guide for the gift they brought you today... wiggle your toes... coming back to the moment... opening your eyes... feeling rejuvenated, tranquil, and balanced...

- **Meridian Balance:** Large Intestine, Kidney, Bladder
- **Musical Note**: Do, C [Vowel Sound U ooh]
- **Reiki Hand Positions**: Base of your body (hold or hover above)
- **Rewrite your Script**: Many of us have painful memories in our past that still pop out of nowhere and cause us stress. It is time that you rewrite that part of your life. *Your subconscious mind (Inner Genie) has no ability to tell imaginary or real apart. Your mind accepts everything as facts until you create an extremely positive or extremely negative emotion in the memory. Rewrite your memory with as*

much extreme positive as you can. Keep saying or writing the new belief. The more you do, the more that becomes your reality.

Change the memory – rewrite it to how you would like it.
- o Anything to do with yourself, finances, home, survival, basic needs

- **Self-Healing:**
    - o Weeding the garden,
    - o Enjoying the fragrances of nature,
    - o Visualizing oneself in a cave during meditation,
    - o Working with clay,
    - o Hugging a tree or leaning back against one,
    - o Lying in the grass,
    - o Crying,
    - o Screaming,
    - o Letting go of inner tensions.
- **Sense:** is anything to do with 'Smell.'

Sacral Chakra

Also Known As – Spleen or Sexx Chakra

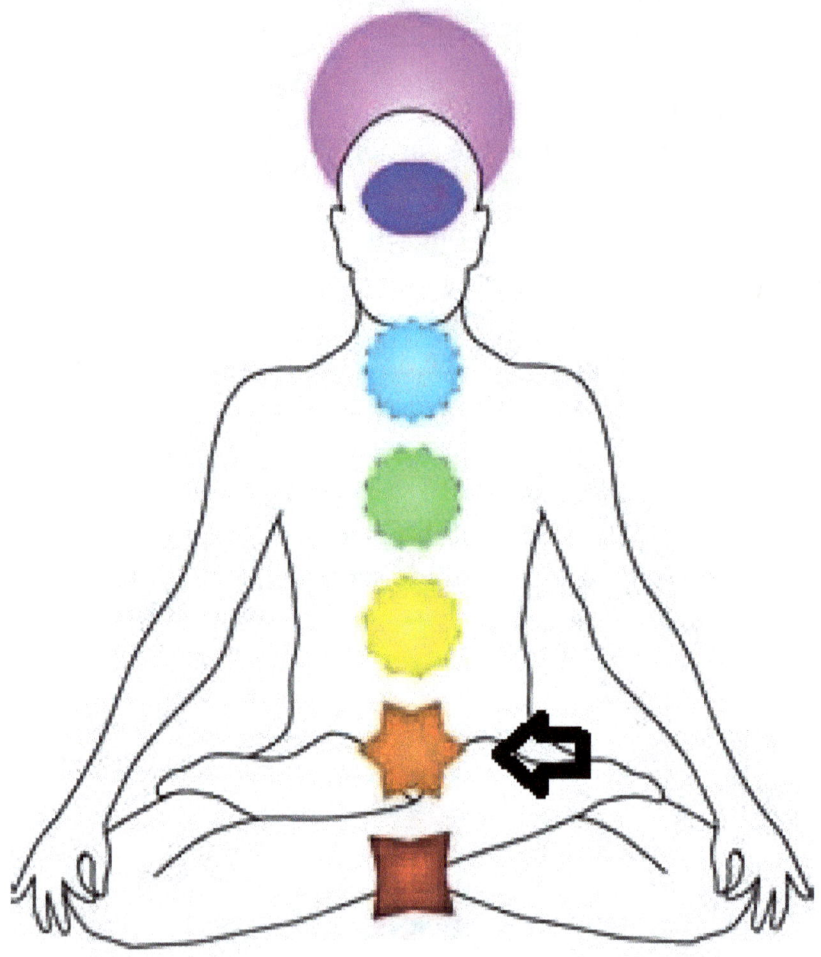

Sanskrit Name Is: Svadhishthana
The Sanskrit name translates to 'one's own.'

Symbol: Sacral Chakra

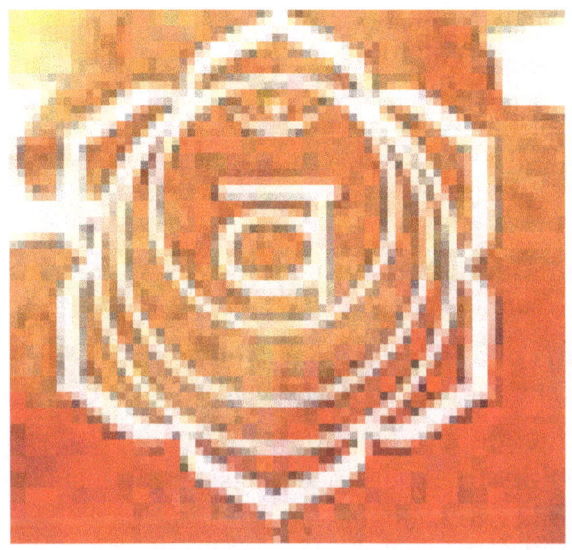

Color in the Rainbow: Orange

Hertz Frequency: 417 Hz

Location: 2nd of the 7 Chakras is:
- Between root Chakra and belly button
- It opens forward and backward

Fundamental Meaning: Happiness, Confidence & Resourcefulness
- Dominate Feelings – Sexuality, Love & Lust
- Pleasure
- All About Them
- Creativity/Sexuality

It is associated with our connection to other people, creativity, energy, confidence, and sexual health.

Organs & Glands controlled by the Sacral Chakra

- Organs,
    - Prostate
    - Kidney (left)
    - Uterus
- Gland
    - Testes or ovaries

Quantum Medicine: Physical Body

Symptoms of a Balanced Sacral Chakra:
Vibrating Good Health & Homeostasis
- Graceful movement
- Ability to experience pleasure & sensuality
- Ability to change
- Ability to nurture self and others
- Creativity
- Enthusiasm for life

Symptoms of PHYSICAL Imbalances of an Under or Over-Balanced Sacral Chakra
Dis-ease:
- Frequent and painful urination
- Cough or sneeze and lose water
- Gout
- Menstruation Issues
- Pre-menstrual syndrome.
- Problems with menstrual flow
- Uterine fibroids.
- Ovarian cysts.
- Endometriosis.
- Testicular disease
- Impotence.

- Prostatic disease.
- Low back pain

Symptoms of EMOTIONAL & MENTAL Imbalances of an Under or Over-Balanced Sacral Chakra
Dis-ease:
- Guilt
- Emotionally sensitive
- Poor boundaries
- Repression,
- Obsessive attachment
- Masked Persona,
- Inhibitions,
- Control,
- Holding onto old relationships

If the sacral (spleen/sexx) Chakra becomes unbalanced, you may feel abandoned, alone, and overwhelmed by family or friends. An imbalanced Sacral Chakra can cause great tribal issues.

Symptoms of SPIRITUAL Imbalances of an Under or Over-Balanced Sacral Chakra
- Not able to feel creative energy from your God source

How to Balance the Sacral Chakra – Body, Mind & Soul

- **Affirmations:**
    - My family loves me just as I am
    - I love the tribe I attract
    - I am truly blessed with my family and friends
    - I have a great sex life
    - I love my body

- Aromatherapy: Melissa, Orange Oil, Damiana, Gardenia, Sandalwood, Ylang-Ylang
- **Communication:** 100% giving
- **Color:** Orange. Immerse yourself in orange-orange clothes, orange foods, orange oils, orange herbs, orange gemstones, orange lights, orange candles, orange flowers, drinking water out of orange glasses, (see the color, wear the color, draw with the color, think the color, taste the color, smell the color, and hear the color)
- **Crystals:** Rhodochrosite, Carnelian, Jasper, Agate, Carnelian, Coral, Moonstone
- **Hertz:** 288 Hz, Tuning Forks, Biofeedback
- **Incense:** Ylang-ylang, Jasmine
- **Meditation - Orange Candle:** Represent happiness and creativity

IDEAS

1) Light an orange candle and stare at the flame. Let your mind go for 2 – 5 minutes.
2) Go to my Constance Santego YouTube Channel to watch and listen to the Sacral Chakra Meditation.
3) Have someone read you this meditation. Find a comfortable place to sit or lie down.

Sacral Chakra Meditation:

Slowly breathe deeply through your nose.
Let all outside noises disappear... release the tension of the muscles in your feet... breathe in and out... relaxing... relax your calves, knees, thighs, and hips... Breathe in and out... relax even more... let go of all the tension in your lower body... breathe in and out... slowly...

As you relax more and more, you start to feel yourself sinking deeper and deeper... Feeling totally safe and secure... Now visualize yourself somewhere in the world... in perfect surroundings, whether it be inside or by an ocean, lake, meadow, or in the mountains... feeling secure...

Look around and see which angel or guide greets you today. Acknowledge each one. Feel their love radiate as an orangish glow penetrates every cell of your being... filling you with creativity, pleasure, and sensuality... Imagine seeing your angel or guide looking lovingly down at you. Sense their smile as a kiss of sunshine from Heaven... healing you from the inside out... Know that they will never let you down. They are a part of you and will always protect you...

Approach your angel or guide with a hug, kiss, or high-five... Enjoy the sensation... Feel the love and warmth... Take as much time as you need to get to know one another...

Feel the trust and bond between the two of you... They tell you they have a specific gift to enhance this Chakra for you... Allow your angel or guide to give it to you... Examine it... feel it, smell it, admire the color and shape... If it is appropriate, even taste it...

Thank your angel or guide and tell them you will always treasure your gift...

It is yours to keep and recall when you feel abandoned or alone... As you hold your gift, feel the love channeled into your Sacral Chakra... Focus on the smooth motion of the Chakra rotating in a clockwise or counterclockwise direction... Feel the warm orange glow that fills the base of your hips... flowing down your legs, calves, and into your feet... this orange energy flows through you into the ground and the earth... Grounding you... and connecting you to your family, friends, and community. Enjoy the wonderful sensation of being blessed by your angels and guides before bringing your attention back to your everyday surroundings…

Take a deep breath and thank your angel or guide for the gift they brought you today… wiggle your toes… coming back to the moment… opening your eyes… feeling rejuvenated, tranquil, and balanced…

- **Meridian Balance:** Kidney, Circulation/Sex or Pericardium
- **Musical Note:** Re, D [Vowel Sound O (home).
- **Reiki Hand Positions:** Back and front of the belly button.
- **Rewrite your Script:** Change the memory – rewrite it to how you would like it to be,
    - Anything to do with your family, friends, community, tribe
- **Self- Healing**
    - Healing baths with apple cider vinegar and Epsom salts,
    - Healing teas (jasmine, hibiscus, chamomile, orange spice),
    - Walking in the rain,
    - Drinking water,
    - Connecting with earth elements,
    - Being silly,
    - Having a personal party.

SECRET OF A HEALER – MAGIC OF REIKI 51

- **Sense:** is anything to do with 'Taste,'

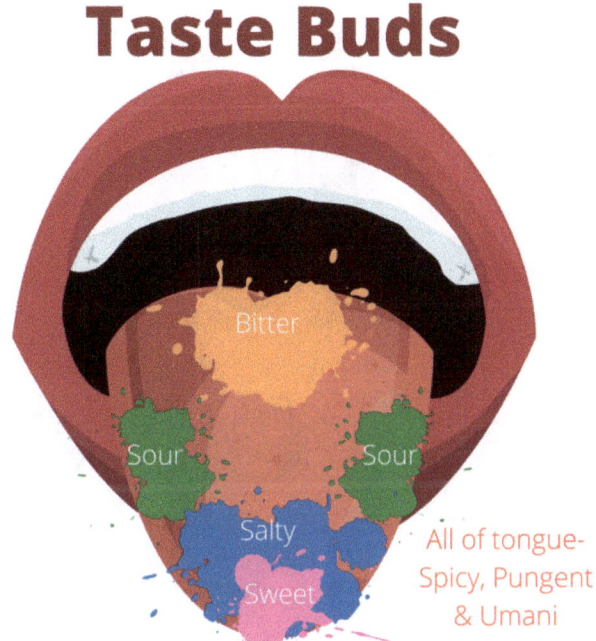

Solar Plexus Chakra

Also Known As – Navel Chakra

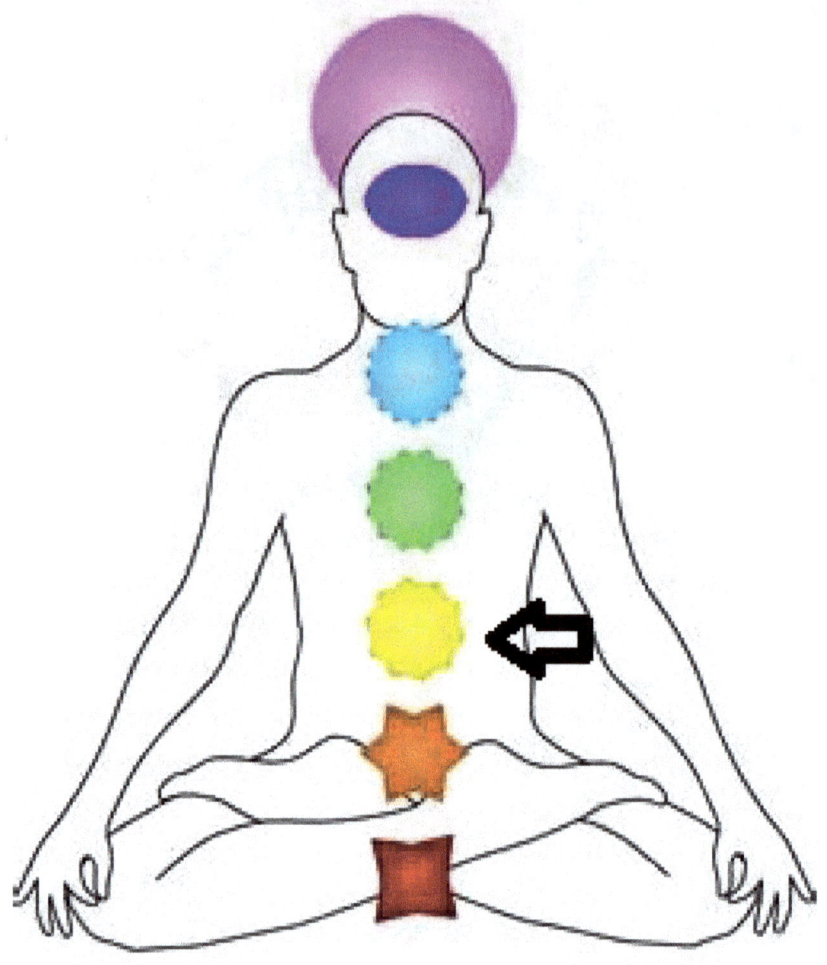

Sanskrit Name Is: Manipura
The Sanskrit name translates to 'lustrous gem.'

Symbol: Solar Plexus Chakra

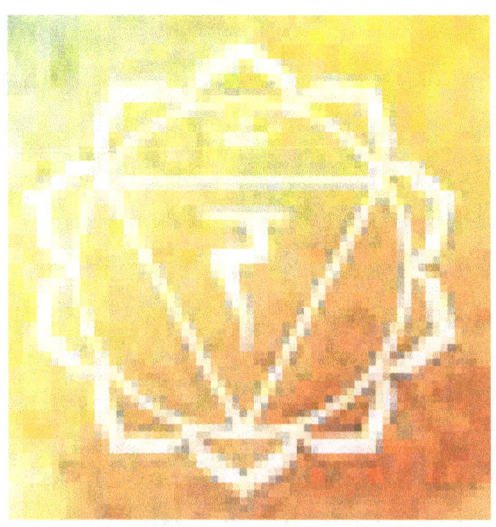

Color in the Rainbow: Yellow

Hertz Frequency: 528 Hz

Location: 3rd of the 7 Chakras is:
- Between the belly button and sternum
- It opens forward and backward

Fundamental Meaning: Wisdom, Clarity & Self-Esteem
- Dominate Feelings – Pride & Unworthiness
- Strength Energy Source
- Will Power, Personal Power, Empowerment

It is associated with our physical center, personal power, will power, desire, inner strength, instincts, and 'gut' feelings.

Organs & Glands controlled by the Solar Plexus Chakra

- Organs,
  - Stomach
  - Spleen
  - Pancreas
  - Liver
  - Gallbladder
  - Small Intestine
- Gland
  - Pancreas

Quantum Medicine: Vital Body

Symptoms of a Balanced Solar Plexus Chakra:
Vibrating Good Health & Homeostasis
- Responsible and reliable,
- Courageous, Empowered & Motivated,
- Confidence and self-esteem,
- Spontaneity, playfulness, and a sense of humor,
- Ability to meet challenges,
- Feeling of peace, balance, and inner harmony,
- Warm personality

Symptoms of PHYSICAL Imbalances of an Under or Over-Balanced Solar Plexus Chakra
Dis-ease:
- Diabetes,
- Jaundice,
- Gallstones,
- Gas pain,
- Indigestion,
- MS,
- Pancreatitis,
- Liver disease,

- Gastric & Peptic ulcers,
- Celica's disease,
- Irritable Bowel,
- Hiatus hernia

Symptoms of EMOTIONAL & MENTAL Imbalances of an Under or Over-Balanced Solar Plexus Chakra Dis-ease:
- Shame,
- Worry,
- Becoming a Follower,
- Power Seeker

Symptoms of Spiritual Imbalances of an Under or Over-Balanced Solar Plexus Chakra Dis-ease;
- Not able to be empowered by your God-source messages

How to Balance the Solar Plexus Chakra – Body, Mind & Soul

- **Affirmations:**
    - I use my willpower appropriately
    - I am powerful
    - I have the energy to spare
    - I act on my inner wisdom
    - My inner strength guides me
- **Aromatherapy:** Rosemary, fennel, bergamot, grapefruit, lemon, lemongrass, petitgrain, marigold.
- **Communication:** Spirit
- **Color:** Yellow. Immerse yourself in yellow - yellow clothes, yellow foods, yellow oils, yellow

herbs, yellow gemstones, yellow lights, yellow candles, yellow flowers, drinking water out of yellow glasses . . . (see the color, wear the color, draw with the color, think the color, taste the color, smell the color, and hear the color)
- **Crystals:** Malachite, Amber, Citrine, Tigers Eye, Topaz, Yellow Sapphire.
- **Hertz:** 320 Hz, Tuning Forks, Biofeedback
- **Incense:** Bergamot, Ginger
- **Meditation - Yellow Candle:** Represent intellect and joy.

IDEAS

4) Light a yellow candle and stare at the flame. Let your mind go for 2 – 5 minutes.
5) Go to my Constance Santego YouTube Channel to watch and listen to the Solar Plexus Chakra Meditation.
6) Have someone read you this meditation. Find a comfortable place to sit or lie down.

Solar Plexus Chakra Meditation:

Slowly breathe deeply through your nose.
Let all outside noises disappear... release the tension of the muscles in your feet... breathing in and out... relaxing... relaxing your calves, knees, and thighs... breathe in and out... relax even more... letting go of all the tension in your stomach... breathe in and out... slowly...

As you relax, you start to feel yourself sinking deeper and deeper... Feeling totally safe and secure... Now visualize yourself somewhere in the world... in perfect surroundings... whether inside or by water, a meadow, or in the mountains... feeling safe and secure...

Look around and see which angel or guide greets you today. Acknowledge each one. Feel their love radiate as a yellowish glow penetrates every cell of your being...

filling you with courage, empowerment, and motivation... Imagine seeing your angel or guide looking lovingly down at you. Sense their smile as a kiss of sunshine from Heaven... healing you from the inside out... Know that they will never let you down. They are a part of you and will always protect you...

Approach your angel or guide with a hug, kiss, or high-five... Enjoy the sensation... Feel the love and warmth... Take as much time as you need to get to know one another...

Feel the trust and bond between the two of you... They tell you they have a specific gift to enhance this Chakra for you... Allow your angel or guide to give it to you... Examine it... feel it, smell it, admire the color and shape... If it is appropriate, even taste it...

Thank your angel or guide and tell them you will always treasure your gift...

It is yours to keep and recall it whenever you feel worried or nervous... As you hold your gift, feel the love being channeled into your Solar Plexus Chakra... Focus the smooth motion of the Chakra rotating in a clockwise or counterclockwise direction... Feel the warm yellow glow that fills your stomach... flowing through and down your hips, legs, calves, and feet... this yellow energy flows through you into the ground and the earth... Grounding you... and connecting you to your inner genie. Enjoy the wonderful sensation of being blessed by your angels and guides before bringing your attention back to your everyday surroundings...

Take a deep breath and thank your angel or guide for the gift they brought to you today... wiggle your toes... coming back to the moment... opening your eyes... feeling rejuvenated, tranquil, and balanced...

- **Meridian Balance:** Stomach, Spleen/Pancreas, Liver, Gallbladder, and Small Intestine
- Kidney, Circulation/Sex, or Pericardium
- **Musical Note:** Mi, E & Eb (Vowel Sound Awh)
- **Reiki Hand Positions:** Back and front of bellybutton
- **Rewrite your Script**: Change the memory – rewrite it to how you would like it to be.
    - Anything to do with your willpower, anger, fear, or get-up-and-go
- **Self-Healing:**
    - Be around friends and loved ones; do things that make you happy and confident.
- **Sense**: is anything to do with 'Sight.'

Heart Chakra

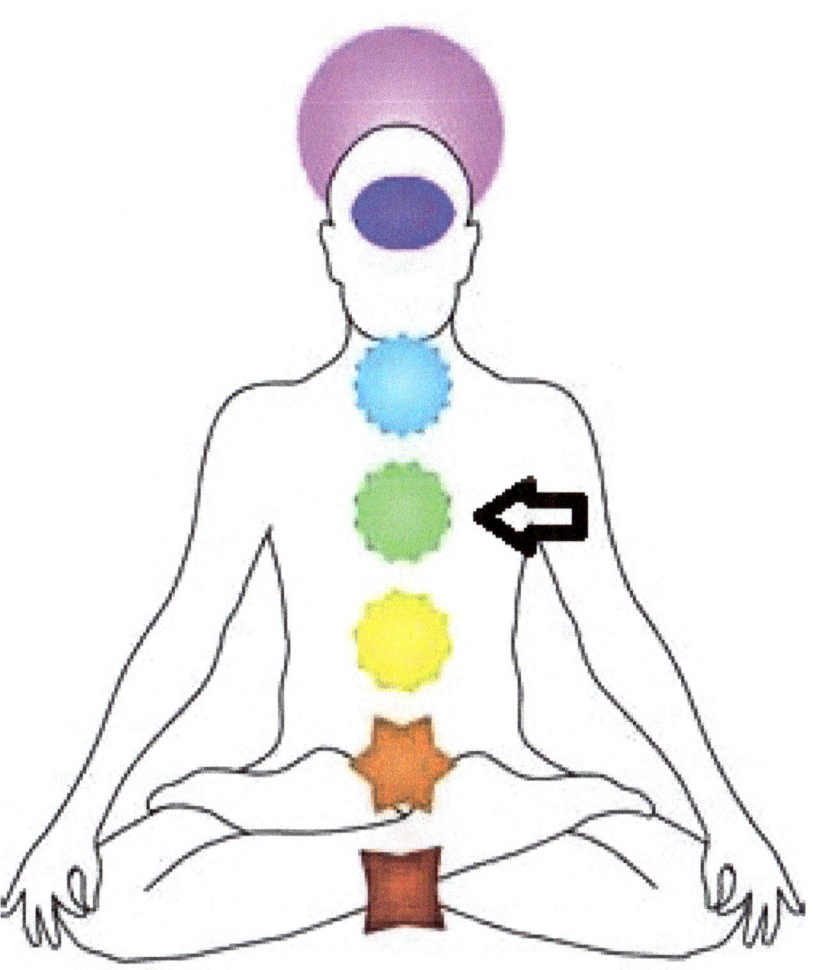

Sanskrit Name Is: Anahata
The Sanskrit name translates to 'unstruck, unhurt, or unbeaten.'

Symbol: Heart Chakra

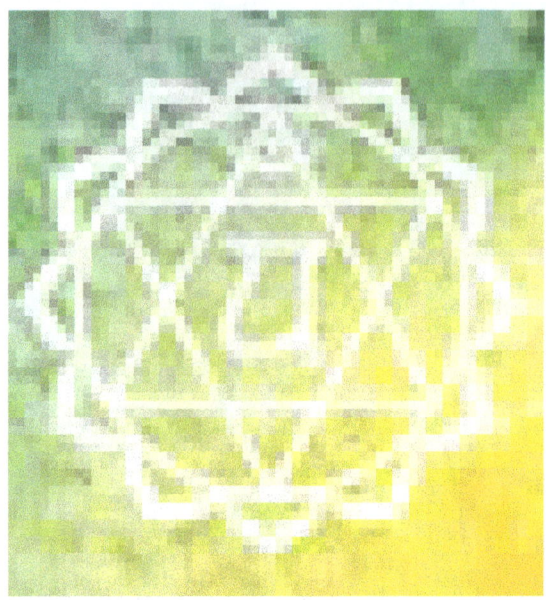

Color in the Rainbow: Green

Hertz Frequency: 639 Hz

Location: 4th of the 7 Chakras is:
- On the sternum
- It opens forward and backward

Fundamental Meaning: Balance, Love & Self-Control
- Dominate Feelings – Romance & Jealousy
- Love Energy Source
- Unites
- Pure Love Connection

It is associated with love, compassion, joy, trust, self-compassion, forgiveness, and relationships.

Organs & Glands controlled by the Heart Chakra

- Organs,
    - Heart
    - Lung
    - Immunity
- Gland
    - Thymus

Quantum Medicine: Vital Body

Symptoms of a Balanced Heart Chakra:
Vibrating Good Health & Homeostasis
- Love & Gratitude
- Warmth, sincerity, and happiness
- A strong connection to all of life
- Compassion
- Willingness to help others
- Peaceful and balanced

Symptoms of PHYSICAL Imbalances of an Under or Over-Balanced Heart Chakra
Dis-ease:

- Blood pressure problems,
- Heart palpitations,
- Blood clots,
- Chest pain
- Blood Pressure
- Heartburn
- Tight Muscles/Cramps & Numbing
- Cancer of the breast
- Diseases of the Immune System, for example, Aids and ME (myalgia, encephalomyelitis, chronic fatigue syndrome, or post-viral syndrome).
- Allergies

Symptoms of EMOTIONAL & MENTAL Imbalances of an Under or Over-Balanced Heart Chakra

- Grief,
- Dissatisfaction,
- Greed,
- Envy,
- Inconsideration,
- Coldness,
- Needing recognition and confirmation from others
- Self-doubting and always blaming others
- Wanting to possess love

Symptoms of SPIRITUAL Imbalances of an Under or Over-Balanced Heart Chakra
Dis-ease;
- Not able to sense the love from your God source

How to Balance the Heart Chakra – Body, Mind & Soul

- **Affirmations:**
    - I love myself
    - I love others
    - Others love me
    - I am happy, content, and fulfilled
    - My heart emanates love and light
- **Aromatherapy:** Eucalyptus, Pine Oil, Marjoram, Orrisroot, Rose Oil, Yarrow
- **Communication:** Feeler
- **Color:** Green. Immerse yourself in green - green clothes, green foods, green oils, green herbs, green gemstones, green lights, green candles, green flowers, drinking water out of green glasses . . . (see the color, wear the color, draw with the color,

think the color, taste the color, smell the color, and hear the color)
- **Crystals:** Moss Agate, Carnelian, Malachite, Emerald, Green Jade, Rose Quartz
- **Hertz:** 341.3 Hz, Tuning Forks, Biofeedback
- **Incense:** Sandalwood, Rose
- Meditation - **Green Candle:** Represent growth and healing.

IDEAS

7) Light a green candle and stare at the flame. Let your mind go for 2 – 5 minutes.
8) Go to my Constance Santego YouTube Channel to watch and listen to the Heart Chakra Meditation.
9) Have someone read you this meditation. Find a comfortable place to sit or lie down.

Heart Chakra Meditation:

Slowly breathe deeply through your nose.
Let all outside noises disappear... release the tension of the muscles in your feet... breathing in and out... relaxing... relaxing your calves, knees, and thighs... breathe in and out... relax even more... letting go of all the tension in your chest... breathe in and out... slowly...

As you relax, you start to feel yourself sinking deeper and deeper... Feeling totally safe and secure... Now visualize yourself somewhere in the world... in perfect surroundings... whether inside or by water, a meadow, or in the mountains... feeling safe and secure...

Look around and see which angel or guide greets you today. Acknowledge each one. Feel their love radiate as a greenish glow penetrates every cell of your being... filling you with love, happiness, and gratitude... Imagine seeing your angel or guide looking lovingly down at you. Sense their smile as a kiss of sunshine from Heaven... healing you from the inside out... Know that they will never let you down. They are a part of you and will always protect you...

Approach your angel or guide with a hug, kiss, or high-five... Enjoy the sensation... Feel the love and warmth... Take as much time as you need to get to know one another...

Feel the trust and bond between the two of you... They tell you they have a specific gift to enhance this Chakra for you... Allow your angel or guide to give it to you... Examine it... feel it, smell it, admire the color and shape... If it is appropriate, even taste it...

Thank your angel or guide and tell them you will always treasure your gift...

It is yours to keep and recall it whenever you feel envy or dissatisfaction... As you hold your gift, feel the love channeled into your Heart Chakra... Focus on the smooth motion of the Chakra rotating in a clockwise or counterclockwise direction... Feel the warm green glow that fills your chest... flowing through and down your rib cage, stomach, hips, legs, calves, and into your feet... this green energy flows through you into the ground and the earth... Grounding you... and connecting you to self-love, compassion, and sincerity. Enjoy the wonderful sensation of being blessed by your angels and guides before bringing your attention back to your everyday surroundings...

Take a deep breath and thank your angel or guide for the gift they brought to you today... wiggle your toes... coming back to the moment... opening your eyes... feeling rejuvenated, tranquil, and balanced...

- **Meridian Balance:** Heart and Lung
- **Musical Note:** Fa, F (Vowel Sound Ah)
- **Reiki Hand Positions:** Back and front of the chest
- **Rewrite your Script:** Change the memory – rewrite it to how you would like it to be.
    - Anything to do with love, relationships, emotions

- **Self-Healing:**
    - Be with nature, feel peace and change within, hug someone or a teddy bear, walk in the wind, and breathe deeply.
- **Sense:** is anything to do with 'Touch.'

Throat Chakra

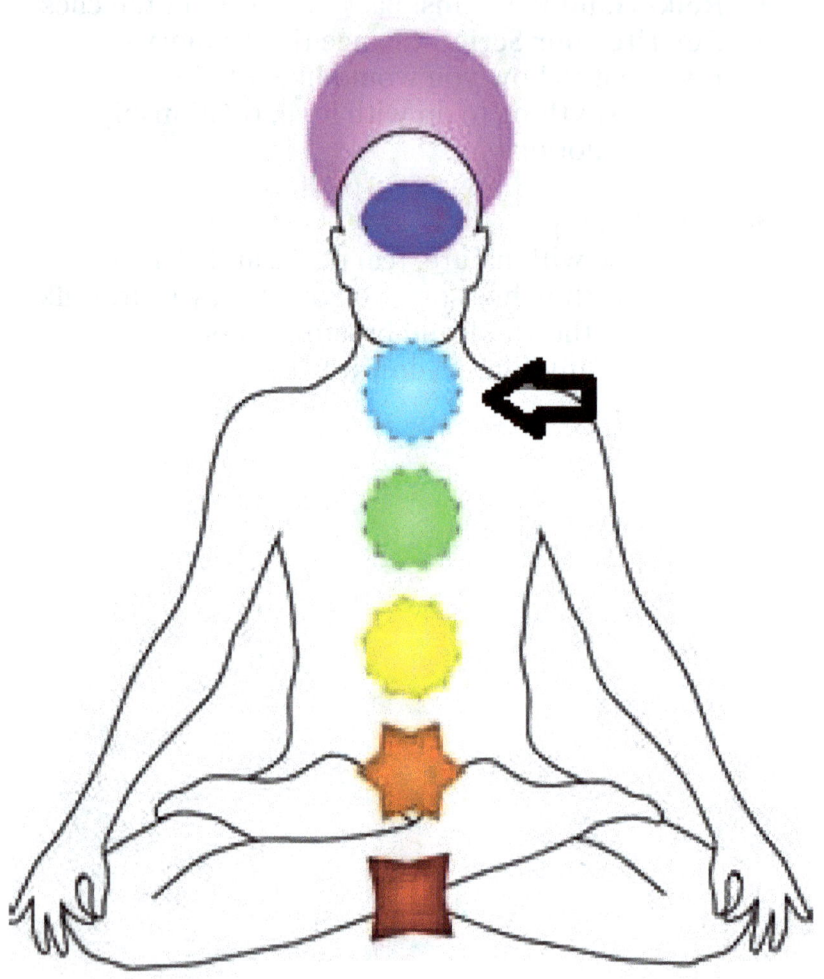

Sanskrit Name Is: Vishuddha
The Sanskrit name translates to 'pure or purification.'

Symbol: Throat Chakra

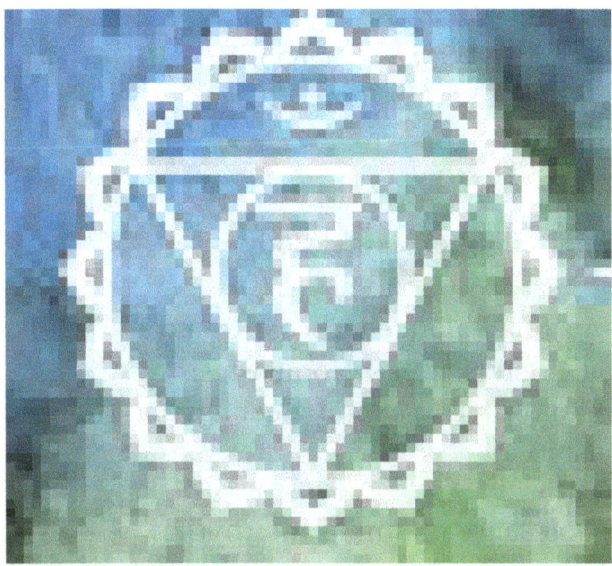

Color in the Rainbow: Blue

Hertz Frequency: 741 Hz

Location: 5th of the 7 Chakras is:
- The throat and neck area
- It opens forward and backward

Fundamental Meaning: Knowledge, Health & Communication
- Dominate Feelings – Exultation & Frustration
- Communication Energy Source
- Verbal Expression
- Truth

It is associated with communication, expression, freedom, responsibility, and leadership.

Organs & Glands controlled by the Throat Chakra

- Organs,
    - Throat & Speech Organs
    - Lungs (Volume Voice)
- Gland
    - Thyroid

Quantum Medicine: Mental Body

Symptoms of a Balanced Throat Chakra:
Vibrating Good Health & Homeostasis
- Openly able to express feelings and thought
- Inspired
- Truth
- Good sense of timing and rhythm
- Imaginative, colorful, and clear speech
- Trusting your inner guidance
- Openly passing knowledge

Symptoms of PHYSICAL Imbalances of an Under or Over-Balanced Throat Chakra
Dis-ease:
- Coughing
- Allergies
- Asthma
- Stuffy nose
- Anorexia nervosa
- Asthma.
- Bronchitis.
- Hearing problems
- Tinnitus (tinnitus may also be connected to issues with the Brow Chakra).
- Thyroid problems - overactive/under-active.

- Mouth ulcers
- Sore throats
- Tonsillitis
- Problems with the upper digestive tract

Symptoms of EMOTIONAL & MENTAL Imbalances of an Under or Over-Balanced Throat Chakra Dis-ease:

- Lies
- Withdrawal,
- Hyperventilation,
- Hysteria,
- Being self-concerned,
- Possessiveness,
- Dominating and controlling behavior
- Resisting Change
- Rigidity
- Stubbornness
- Slow to respond

Symptoms of SPIRITUAL Imbalances of an Under or Over-Balanced Throat Chakra Dis-ease:

- Not able to speak or hear the truth from your God source

How to Balance the Throat Chakra – Body, Mind & Soul

- **Affirmations:**
    - I speak my truth
    - I communicate perfectly

- - o I can express myself freely
    - o My inner guidance speaks to me, and I understand
    - o I love to share my knowledge
- **Aromatherapy:** Geranium, Chamomile Oil, Benzoin, Eucalyptus, Frankincense, Sage.
- **Communication:** Audio
- **Color:** Blue. Immerse yourself in blue - blue clothes, blue foods, blue oils, blue herbs, blue gemstones, blue lights, blue candles, blue flowers, drinking water out of blue glasses . . . (see the color, wear the color, draw with the color, think the color, taste the color, smell the color, and hear the color)
- **Crystals:** Amber, Lapis Lazuli, Blue Topaz, Aquamarine, Blue Sapphire
- **Hertz:** 384 Hz, Tuning Forks, Biofeedback
- **Incense:** Frankincense, Peppermint
- **Meditation - Blue Candle:** Represent trust and confidence

IDEAS

1. Light a blue candle and stare at the flame. Let your mind go for 2 – 5 minutes.
2. Go to my Constance Santego YouTube Channel to watch and listen to the Throat Chakra Meditation.
3. Have someone read you this meditation. Find a comfortable place to sit or lie down.

Throat Chakra Meditation:

Slowly breathe deeply through your nose.
Let all outside noises disappear... release the tension of the muscles in your feet... breathe in and out... relax... relaxing your calves, knees, and thighs... breathe in and

out... relax even more... letting go of all the tension in your neck... breathing in and out... slowly...

As you relax, you start to feel yourself sinking deeper and deeper... Feeling safe and secure... Now visualize yourself somewhere in the world... in perfect surroundings... whether inside or by water, in a meadow, or in the mountains... feeling safe and secure...

Look around and see which angel or guide greets you today. Acknowledge each one. Feel their love radiate as a blueish glow penetrates every cell of your being... filling you with inspiration, truth, and expression... Imagine seeing your angel or guide looking lovingly down at you. Sense their smile as a kiss of sunshine from Heaven... healing you from the inside out... Know that they will never let you down. They are a part of you and will always protect you...

Approach your angel or guide with a hug, kiss, or high-five... Enjoy the sensation... Feel the love and warmth... Take as much time as you need to get to know one another...

Feel the trust and bond between the two of you... They tell you they have a specific gift to enhance this Chakra for you... Allow your angel or guide to give it to you... Examine it... feel it, smell it, admire the color and shape... If it is appropriate, even taste it...

Thank your angel or guide and tell them you will always treasure your gift...

It is yours to keep and recall it whenever you feel withdrawn or concerned... As you hold your gift, feel the love being channeled into your Throat Chakra... Focus on the smooth motion of the Chakra rotating in a clockwise or counterclockwise direction... Feel the soothing blue glow that fills your throat... flowing through and down your neck, chest, stomach, hips, legs, calves, and into your feet... this blue energy flows through you into the ground and the earth... Grounding you... connecting you to your passions. Enjoy the incredible sensation of being blessed by your angels and guides before bringing your attention back to your everyday surroundings...

Take a deep breath and thank your angel or guide for the gift they brought to you today... wiggle your toes... coming back to the moment... opening your eyes... feeling rejuvenated, tranquil, and balanced...

- **Meridian Balance:** Lung
- **Musical Note:** Sol, G (Vowel Sound Eh)
- **Reiki Hand Positions:** Back and front of the throat
- **Rewrite your Script**: Change the memory – rewrite it to how you would like it to be.
    - Anything to do with communication, singing, talking, listening, writing, and reading.
- **Self-Healing:**
    - Chanting, singing, whistling, yelling, screaming, laughing, and singing in the shower.
- **Sense:** is anything to do with 'Sound.'

Brow Chakra

Also Known As – Third Eye Chakra

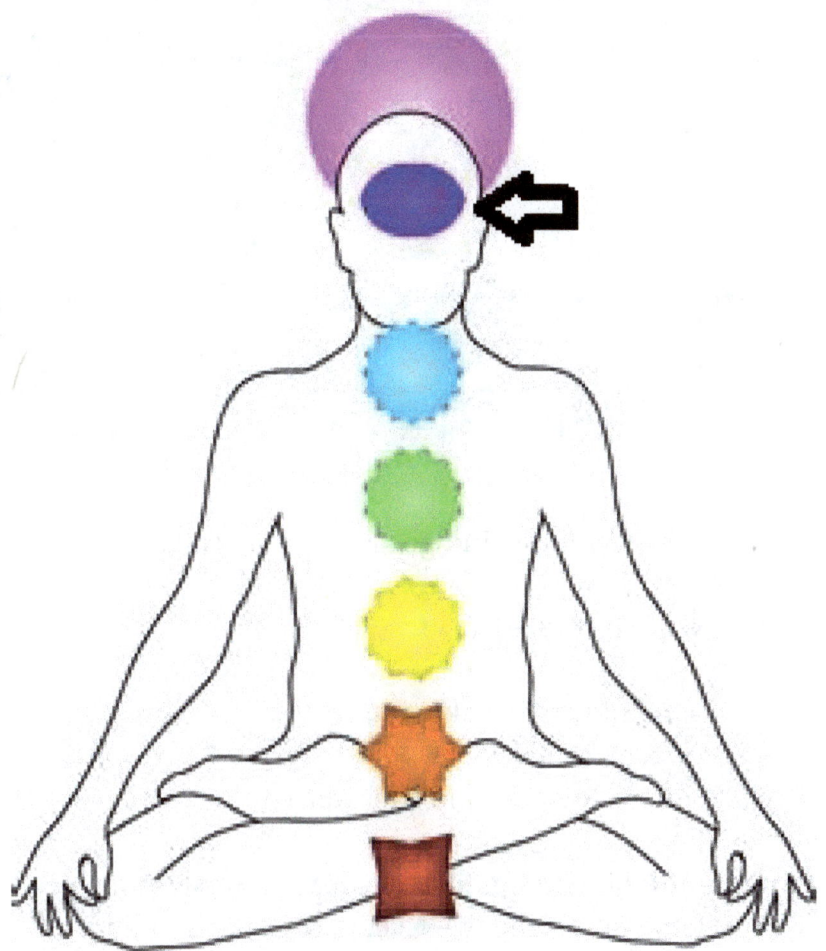

Sanskrit Name Is: Ajna
The Sanskrit name translates to 'perceive, command, or beyond wisdom.'

Symbol: Brow Chakra

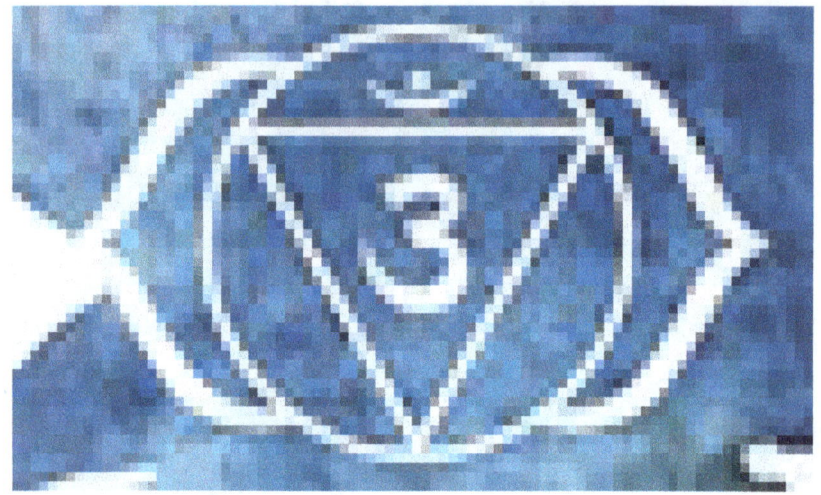

Color in the Rainbow: Indigo

Hertz Frequency: 852 Hz

Location: 6th of the 7 Chakras is:
- Between the eyebrows
- It opens forward and backward

Fundamental Meaning: Mysticism & Understanding
- Dominate Feelings – Clarity & Confusion
- Six Sense/Intuition Energy Source
- Insight

It is associated with the mind, ideas, thoughts, dreams, intuition, and psychic abilities.

Organs & Glands are controlled by the Brow Chakra

- Organs,
    - Hindbrain
    - Midbrain
    - Eyes
    - Autonomic Nervous System
- Gland
    - Pituitary

Quantum Medicine: Supramental Body

Symptoms of a Balanced Brow Chakra:
Vibrating Good Health & Homeostasis
- Insight & Imagery
- Intuitive and Perceptive
- Imaginative
- Live & think holistically
- Advanced intellectual skills

Symptoms of PHYSICAL Imbalances of an Under or Over-Balanced Brow Chakra
Dis-ease:
- Sleep disturbances
- Concentration
- Headaches
- Tension headache
- Migraine
- Disorders of the eyes, visual defects
- Short-sightedness
- Long-sightedness
- Glaucoma
- Cataract.
- Catarrh
- Some ear or sinuses problems

- Endocrine imbalances (because of the association with the pituitary gland)

Symptoms of EMOTIONAL & MENTAL Imbalances of an Under or Over-Balanced Brow Chakra Dis-ease:
- Illusion
- Not wanting to see something important for spiritual growth,
- Worrying
- Fear of Future
- Forgetful
- Over-sensitivity
- Arrogance,
- Obsession,
- Neurotic behavior,
- Pretension,
- Loftiness

Symptoms of SPIRITUAL Imbalances of an Under or Over-Balanced Brow Chakra Dis-ease:
- Not able to use your psychic or intuitive abilities from your God source

How to Balance the Brow Chakra – Body, Mind & Soul

- **Affirmations:**
    - My perceptions are accurate
    - I trust my gut instincts
    - I am imaginatively creative
    - I believe in what I sense

- o I follow my intuition
- **Aromatherapy**: Jasmine, Mint, Mugwort, Star Anise
- **Communication:** Visual
- **Color:** Indigo/Cobalt Blue. Immerse yourself in indigo - indigo clothes, indigo foods, indigo oils, indigo herbs, indigo gemstones, indigo lights, indigo candles, indigo flowers, and drinking water out of indigo glasses . . . (see the color, wear the color, draw with the color, think the color, taste the color, smell the color, and hear the color)
- **Crystals:** Azurite/Silver - place amethyst on the brow/third eye area for soothing
- **Hertz:** 426.7 Hz, Tuning Forks, Biofeedback
- **Incense:** Cinnamon, Sage
- Meditation - **Indigo Candle:** Represent higher consciousness and inner wisdom.

IDEAS

1. Light an indigo candle and stare at the flame. Let your mind go for 2 – 5 minutes.
2. Go to my Constance Santego YouTube Channel to watch and listen to the Brow Chakra Meditation.
3. Have someone read you this meditation. Find a comfortable place to sit or lie down.

Brow Chakra Meditation:

Slowly breathe deeply through your nose.
Let all outside noises disappear... release the tension of the muscles in your feet... breathing in and out... relaxing... relaxing your calves, knees, and thighs... breathe in and out... relax even more... letting go of all the tension in your forehead... breathe in and out... slowly...

As you relax more, you start to feel yourself sinking deeper and deeper... Feeling safe and secure... Now visualize yourself somewhere in the world... in perfect surroundings... whether inside or by water, a meadow, or in the mountains... feeling safe and secure...

Look around and see which angel or guide greets you today. Acknowledge each one. Feel their love radiate as a cobalt-blueish glow penetrates every cell of your being... filling you with insight, imagery, and intuition... Imagine seeing your angel or guide looking lovingly down at you. Sense their smile as a kiss of sunshine from Heaven... healing you from the inside out... Know that they will never let you down. They are a part of you and will always protect you...

Approach your angel or guide with a hug, kiss, or high-five... Enjoy the sensation... Feel the love and warmth... Take as much time as you need to get to know one another...

Feel the trust and bond between the two of you... They tell you they have a specific gift to enhance this Chakra for you... Allow your angel or guide to give it to you... Examine it... feel it, smell it, admire the color and shape... If it is appropriate, even taste it...

Thank your angel or guide and tell them you will always treasure your gift...

It is yours to keep and recall when you feel arrogance or forgetfulness... As you hold your gift, feel the love channeled into your Brow Chakra... Focus on the smooth motion of the Chakra rotating in a clockwise or counterclockwise direction... Feel the warm indigo glow that fills your face... flowing through and down your forehead, neck, chest, stomach, hips, legs, calves, and into your feet... this indigo energy flows through you into the ground and the earth... Grounding you... and connecting you to your subconscious mind... Enjoy the wonderful sensation of being blessed by your angels and guides before bringing your attention back to your everyday surroundings...

Take a deep breath and thank your angel or guide for the gift they brought to you today... wiggle your toes... coming back to the moment... opening your eyes... feeling rejuvenated, tranquil, and balanced...

- **Meridian Balance:** Sanjiao or Triple Warmer, Ren or Conception Vessel, Du or Governing Vessel
- **Musical Note:** La, A (Vowel Sound Ee)
- **Reiki Hand Positions:** back and front of the throat
- **Rewrite your Script:** Change the memory – rewrite it to how you would like it to be.
    - Anything to do with intuition, psychics, metaphysics
- **Self-Healing:**
    - Meditate on the color indigo blue, visualize the completion of goals, and activate your inner imagery
- **Sense:** is anything to do with 'Color & Light.'

Crown Chakra

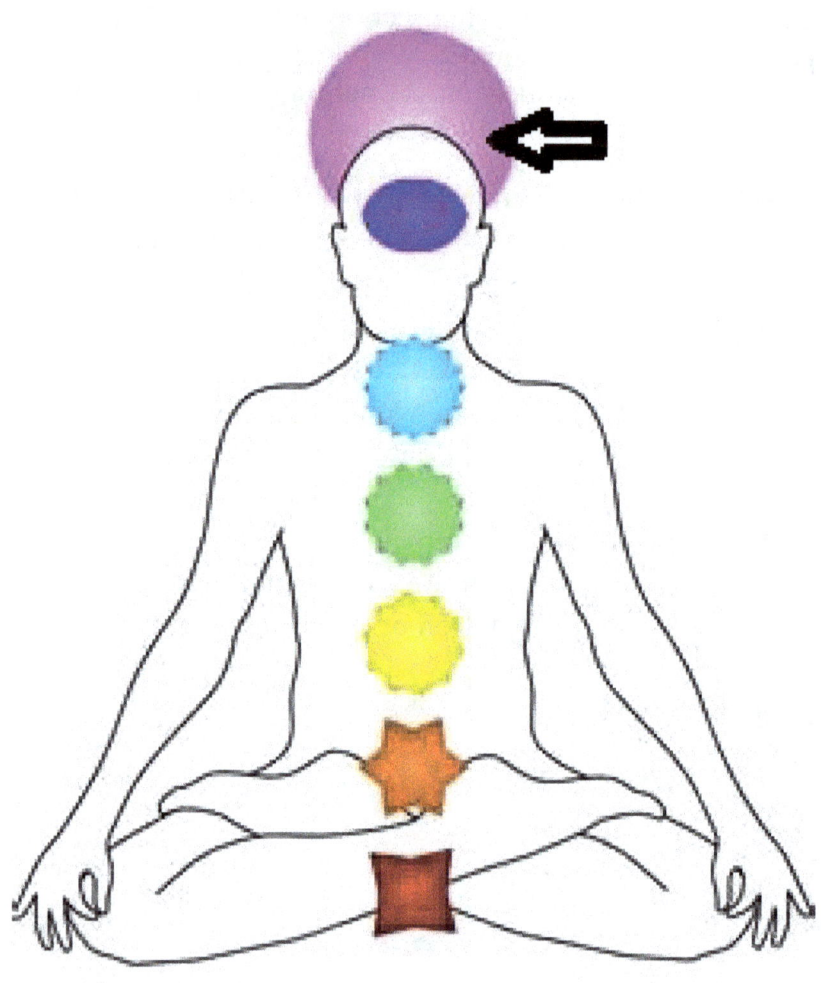

Sanskrit Name Is: **Sahasrara**
The Sanskrit name translates to 'thousand petals.'

Symbol: Crown Chakra

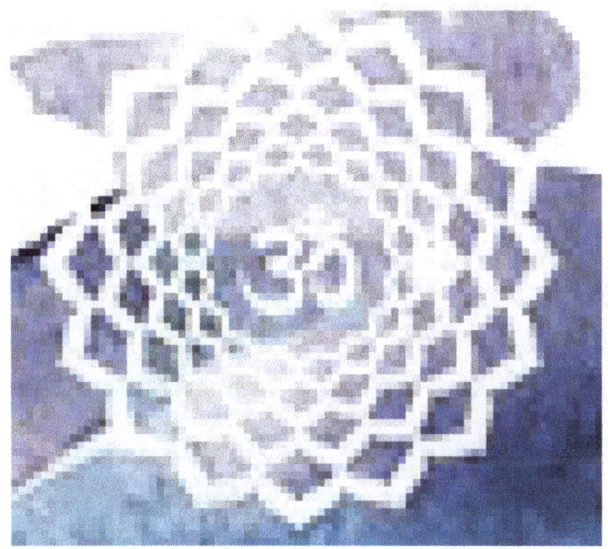

Color in the Rainbow: Violet

Hertz Frequency: 963 Hz

Location: 7th of the 7 Chakras is:
- The baby's soft spot on top of the head
- It opens upward

Fundamental Meaning: Beauty, Creativity & Inspiration
- Dominate Feelings – Satisfaction & Despair
- Cosmic & Spiritual Energy Source
- Enlightenment

It is associated with God (or your belief system), spirituality, divine wisdom, enlightening, connection to the universe, imagination, awareness, and optimism.

Organs & Glands are controlled by the Crown Chakra

- Organs,
    - Neocortex
    - Central Nervous System (CNS)
- Gland
    - Pineal

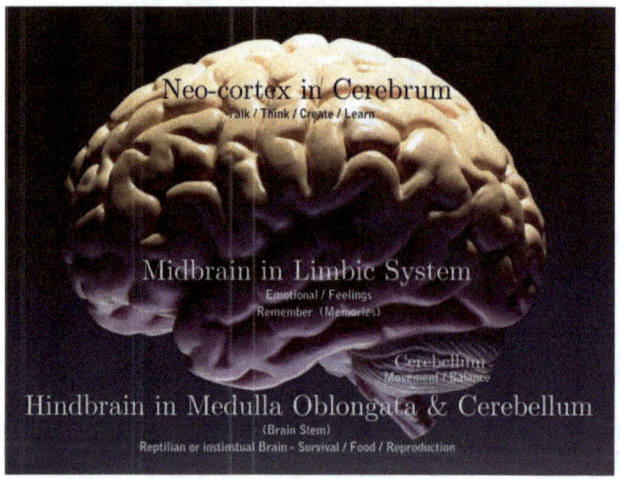

Quantum Medicine: Bliss Body

Symptoms of a Balanced Crown Chakra:
Vibrating Good Health & Homeostasis
- Joy & Bliss
- Intelligent
- Thoughtful and aware
- Open-minded
- Wisdom
- Perception
- Mastery
- Enlightenment

Symptoms of PHYSICAL Imbalances of an Under or Over-Balanced Crown Chakra
Dis-ease:
- Tiredness
- Cerebral dysfunction
- migraines, and nervous tension
- Nervous system
- Poor short-term memory
- Tired
- Parkinson's disease
- Schizophrenia
- Epilepsy
- Senile dementia
- Alzheimer's
- Many mental disorders
- Confusion
- Dizziness, and even just feeling as if one has a muzzy head

Symptoms of EMOTIONAL & MENTAL Imbalances of an Under or Over-Balanced Crown Chakra
Dis-ease:
- Ego
- Need Sympathy
- Shame
- Negative self-image
- Feeling misunderstood
- Psychosis
- Feeling overwrought
- Creative exhaustion

Symptoms of SPIRITUAL Imbalances of an Under or Over-Balanced Crown Chakra
Dis-ease:
- Not able to connect to your God source

How to Balance the Crown Chakra – Body, Mind & Soul

- **Affirmations:**
    - I have faith
    - I connect freely to my God's source
    - My body's wisdom is brilliant
    - I am open to new ideas
    - I am enlightened
- **Aromatherapy:** Lotus, Rose, Spruce
- **Crystals:** Clear Quartz, Fluorite, and Amethyst
- **Communication:** Knower
- **Color:** Indigo/Cobalt Blue. Immerse yourself in indigo - indigo clothes, indigo foods, indigo oils, indigo herbs, indigo gemstones, indigo lights, indigo candles, indigo flowers, and drinking water out of indigo glasses . . . (see the color, wear the color, draw with the color, think the color, taste the color, smell the color, and hear the color)
- **Hertz:** 480 Hz, Tuning Forks, Biofeedback
- **Incense:** Frankincense, Myrrh, Lotus
- **Meditation - Violet Candle:** Represent ambition and luxury.

IDEAS

1. Light a violet candle and stare at the flame. Let your mind go for 2 – 5 minutes.
2. Go to my Constance Santego YouTube Channel to watch and listen to the Crown Chakra Meditation.
3. Have someone read you this meditation. Find a comfortable place to sit or lie down.

Crown Chakra Meditation:

Slowly breathe deeply through your nose.
Let all outside noises disappear... release the tension of the muscles in your feet... breathe in and out... relax... relax your calves, knees, and thighs... breathe in and out... relax even more... let go of all the tension in your head... breathing in and out... slowly...

As you relax, you start to feel yourself sinking deeper and deeper... Feeling totally safe and secure... Now visualize yourself somewhere in the world... in perfect surroundings... whether inside or by water, a meadow, or in the mountains... feeling safe and secure...

Look around and see which angel or guide greets you today. Acknowledge each one. Feel their love radiate as a purplish glow penetrates every cell of your being... filling you with joy, bliss, and enlightenment... Imagine seeing your angel or guide looking lovingly down at you. Sense their smile as a kiss of sunshine from Heaven... healing you from the inside out... Know that they will never let you down. They are a part of you and will always protect you...

Approach your angel or guide with a hug, kiss, or high-five... Enjoy the sensation... Feel the love and warmth... Take as much time as you need to get to know one another...

Feel the trust and bond between the two of you... They tell you they have a specific gift to enhance this Chakra for you... Allow your angel or guide to give it to you... Examine it... feel it, smell it, admire the color and shape... If it is appropriate, even taste it...

Thank your angel or guide and tell them you will always treasure your gift...

It is yours to keep and recall whenever you feel misunderstood or shameful... As you hold your gift, feel the love being channeled into your Crown Chakra... Focus the smooth motion of the Chakra rotating in a clockwise or counterclockwise direction... Feel the warm violet glow that fills your head... flowing through and down your forehead, face, neck, chest, stomach, hips, legs, calves, and into your feet... this violet energy flows through you into the ground and the earth... Grounding you... and connecting you to your God source. Enjoy the wonderful sensation of being blessed by your angels and guides before bringing your attention back to your everyday surroundings...

Take a deep breath and thank your angel or guide for the gift they brought to you today... wiggle your toes... coming back to the moment... opening your eyes... feeling rejuvenated, tranquil, and balanced...

- **Musical Note:** Ti, B (Vowel Sound OHM)
  Rewrite your Script: Change the memory – rewrite it to how you would like it to be.
    - Anything to do with God, Creator, Universe, Angels, and Guides.
- **Reiki Hand Positions:** Back, top, forehead, and sides of the head.
- **Self-Healing:**
    - Dance, music, writing, retreat into nature, and meditation.
- **Sense:** is anything to do with 'Thought.'

PART TWO

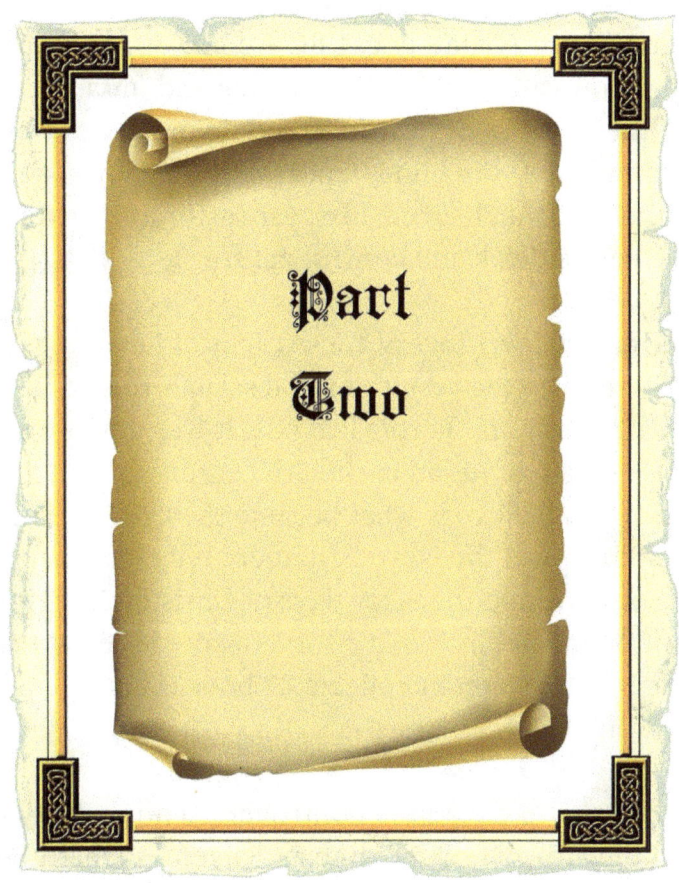

History of Hands-on-Healing

Many of you have heard the stories from the Bible about Jesus, also referred to as Jesus of Nazareth or Jesus Christ (approximately c. 4 BC – c. AD 30/33). There are numerous stories about his healing and miraculous abilities. Stories of how he could do paralytics (faith healing), cure the blind, lepers, bleeding, dropsy, withered hand, hearing loss, ear restoration, exorcism, raising the dead, and control nature.

The original writings of these types of healings were written from the result of royal scribes recording the royal history and heroic legends. It was during the reign of Hezekiah of Judah in the 8th century B.C. that historians believe is what became the Old Testament in the Bible. And the New Testament tells the stories of the life of Jesus and the early days of Christianity. They were written mainly in Paul's efforts to spread Jesus' teaching. The New Testament collects 27 books, all originally written in Greek.

And if you had read the controversial book 'Holy Blood and the Holy Grail' by Michael Baigent, Richard Leigh, and Henry Lincoln, you would have investigated another side of how Jesus learned these metaphysical techniques. It is written that he had learned the "Craft." *Dan Brown's book and movie, 'The Da Vinci Code,' is also on this same basis.*

Another origin of ancient scripture and history was found in the 'Dead Sea Scrolls' (aka Qumran Caves Scrolls). These are ancient Jewish religious manuscripts that were found in the Qumran Caves in the Judaean Desert, near Ein Feshkha on the northern shore of the Dead Sea in the West Bank.

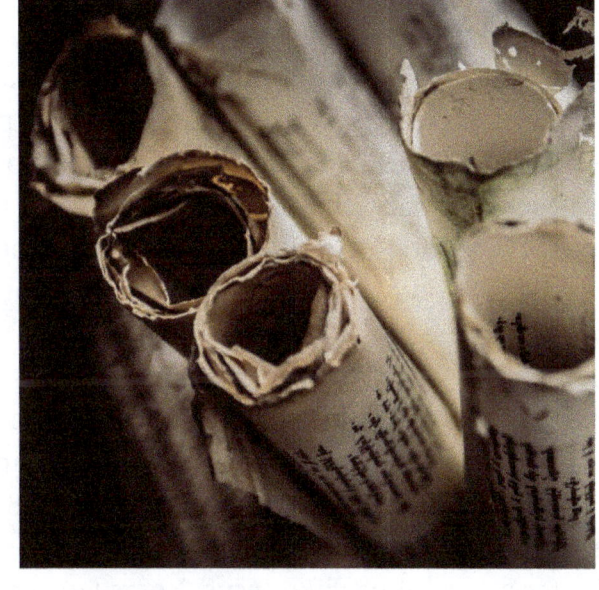

Scholarly consensus dates these scrolls from the last three centuries BCE and the first century CE. It was believed that the Jewish people killed themselves rather than surrender to the Romans. Still, before they did, they wrote about the historical, religious, and linguistic significance and then buried the information so it would not be destroyed.

Book burning is recorded as early as 259–210 B.C. The Chinese emperor Shih Huang Ti burned books so others could not follow the knowledge, as did the Nazi book burning in Berlin in May 1933.

The translation of these Dead Sea Scrolls writings was from the Hebrew language. The collection also included many Aramaic and Greek texts, some Arabic texts, and a small number of Latin fragments.

Healing dates back even further; as far back as Ancient Egypt, Pharaohs believed in magic and the magical power of the written word in healing. Among these protective tools was the 'Horus Magic Paintings,' these paintings were used for many therapeutic purposes. Also, the statue of 'Djedhor,' the healer, had rumors about its power. Even today, many have claimed that it is a magical healing statue.

A more recent account of hands-on-healing healing and miraculous abilities was by an East Indian man, born on 23 November 1926 to Sathyanarayana Raju. By the age of fourteen, he was another human that could perform miracles and healings like Jesus. Years later, he changed his name to Sri Sathya Sai Baba, a guru and philanthropist. Dedicating his life to healing others, he died at age eight-four, 24 April 2011.

Healings by mystical or unexplained power have been around since the beginning of time and are teachable to those that seek its truth.

Dr. Usui's Reiki Method

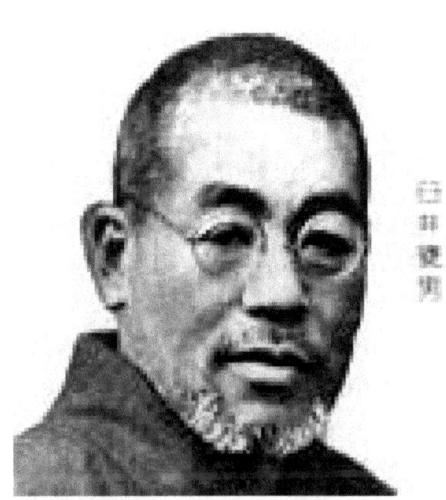

Reiki originated in Tibet and was discovered in the nineteenth century by a Japanese monk, Dr. Mikao Usui was born to a wealthy Buddhist family (15 August 1865 - 9 March 1926).

Dr. Usui's family was able to give their son a well-rounded education for the time. As a child, Dr. Usui studied in a Buddhist monastery where he was taught martial arts, swordsmanship, and the Japanese form of Chi Kung, known as Kiko (Qigong).

Adding to his comprehension of Japanese, Dr. Usui learned Sanskrit and Chinese, as well as other languages, so that he could study each manuscript himself, and nothing would be 'lost' or 'misinterpreted' in translation.

In the mid-1800s, Dr. Mikao Usui was studying the ancient Sanskrit writings and the healing technique of Jesus. Dr. Usui was transfixed in unraveling the secrets of healing. So he went on a quest to find out how Buddha and Jesus had healed with their hands.

He found what he thought would be key to physical healing in the Sanskrit sutras. He discovered symbols, formulas, and intellectual writings but did not find the method or technique.

He asked for advice on what he should do from the Abbott of the Zen Buddhist monastery where he was staying. They decided that he should go to the scared Mount Kurama, outside of Kyoto in the Kuriyama district, which is situated in the central region of Hokkaido. The name *Kuriyama means 'Chestnut Mountain' in Japanese.*

For 21 days, he would fast and meditate to see if he could gain insight into the use of the information that he found. Dr. Usui collected 21 stones to keep track of his time in a cave on the mountain. Each day he threw one stone away and then meditated and fasted.

On the morning of the 21st day, he still had not received the knowledge he sought. As he prayed that morning that before dawn, he would be shown the light and how to use the 'keys to healing' that he had found in the scriptures, he threw away his last stone.

Disappointed that evening for not accomplishing his quest, he stood up to leave, and as he did so, a little beam of light way off on the horizon started to move toward him. As it came closer, it became bigger and bigger, nearly frightening him to death. He had spent years on this quest and was not about to run now. Finally, as he braced himself, the light struck him in the middle of his forehead and knocked him out.

In his dream state, he experienced a rainbow of colors, and the Sanskrit symbols, their use, and meanings were drawn in the sky. In his initial attunement, Dr. Usui received all the keys to healing. He vowed never to forget them or allow them to be lost.

Dr. Usui was ecstatic about his experience and newfound knowledge and quickly started down the mountain back to Kyoto and the monastery. On his journey back, the 'Four Miracles of Reiki' happened.

Miracle number one, in his haste, he tripped and stubbed his toe. He instinctively bent down, held his aching toe between his hands, and soon realized that the pain and bleeding had stopped. He also noticed a great deal of heat-generating out of his hands.

Miracle number two happened when he broke his twenty-one-day fast by ordering a full meal at a home that served travelers. He ate the entire meal and did not suffer any indigestion or discomfort.

Miracle number three, the young girl serving him, suffered from an abscessed tooth. Again, Dr. Usui placed his hands on the swelling, and within moments, the pain and swelling disappeared.

Miracle number four happened back at the monastery. The Abbott was in dire pain from an arthritis attack. Dr. Usui placed his hands on the area of pain while sharing his experiences with the Abbott; very quickly, the pain disappeared.

After much meditation and consulting with the Abbott, Dr. Usui decided to use his new healing knowledge, which he called Reiki, on the poor, diseased, and crippled. So for many years, he worked with these people, giving healing.

But years later, one day, he noticed that many of the people he healed had returned to their lives as beggars. When he asked why, they replied that it was much easier, with no responsibilities.

Frustrated with this and feeling like he had failed, Dr. Usui realized that even though he had healed, he did not teach any responsibility. Therefore, an equal energy exchange, monetary or other, was required from that day forward.

From this experience, Dr. Usui created the 'Five Principles of Reiki.'
Just for Today,
1. I will not worry,
2. I shall do my work honestly,
3. I shall accept my many blessings,
4. I shall deal with anger appropriately,
5. I shall show love and respect for everyone and everything.

In 1922, Dr. Usui *(Usui Sensei -teacher or instructor)* founded his first Reiki clinic and school in Tokyo and taught Reiki. He trained approximately sixteen Reiki Masters. And before his death, he gave Dr. Chujiro

Hayashi the responsibility of preserving and passing on the tradition of Reiki.

It was Dr. Hayashi who developed the three levels of Reiki,

- 1st Degree/Level 1 – Apprentice,
  - Physical Self-healing,
- 2nd Degree/Level 2- Practitioner, Healing others,
  - Body and mind healing,
- 3rd Degree/Level 3 – Master, Teacher – Teaching others
  - Spiritual healing.

As World War II was coming, Dr. Hayashi feared Reiki's survival, knowing that many men would die in the war. So Dr. Hayashi decided to train a Japanese woman living in Hawaii, Mrs. Hawayo Takata.

Mrs. Takata brought Reiki training to the United States and Canada and was the one who decided to charge a fee for each level of training.

Levels of Reiki

FIRST-DEGREE REIKI, LEVEL I – APPRENTICE

Body - All about self-healing!

WHAT DO YOU LEARN?
- 1st degree Reiki Attunement (Meet your Reiki Master in Spirit),
- Reiki Energy,
- Chakras,
- Physical Healing,
- Self-Healing using the seven major Chakras and the 16 minor Chakra hand positions.

SECOND-DEGREE REIKI, LEVEL II – PRACTITIONER

Body & Mind - All about healing ANOTHER person!

WHAT DO YOU LEARN NEW?
- 2nd degree Reiki Attunement,
- Using the hand position of level 1 (7 major Chakras and the 16 minor Chakras) and combining it with 361 Tsubo points on the body,
- Chakra Crystal Healing,
- Chakra Pendulum Healing,
- Mental & Emotional Healing,
- Distance Healing.

THIRD-DEGREE REIKI, LEVEL III – MASTER

Body, Mind & Soul - All about TEACHING another person!

WHAT DO YOU LEARN NEW?
- 3rd degree Reiki Attunement,
- You learned physical healing in Level 1, mental & emotional healing in Level 2, and now in Level 3, you will learn Spiritual Healing,
- PLUS!!! How to teach Reiki to others. You become the Teacher!

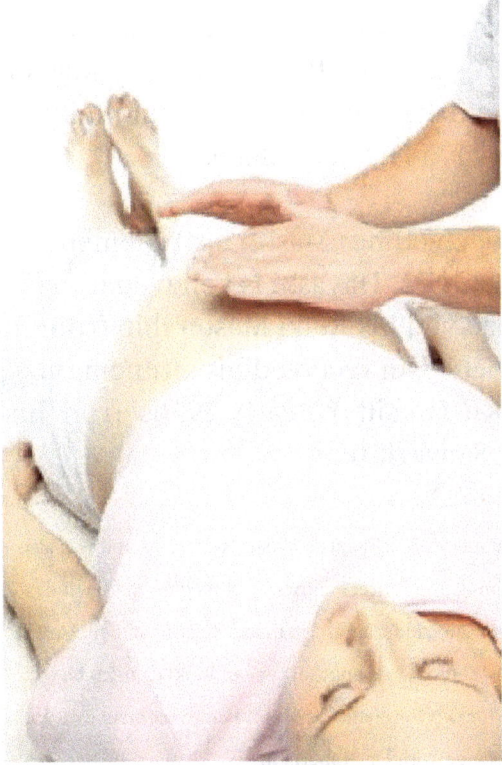

The degree of Reiki does not equate to the amount of energy you have to use.

The degree only refers to the knowledge you learn within each level.

Lineage

I was initiated into Reiki Levels 1 & 2 in September 1999 by an American lady called Nefertiti.

In the year 2010, I, Constance Santego, under the name Connie Brummet, was attuned to Grand Reiki Mastery by Spirit, BUT in 2000, I was attuned to Reiki Mastery by Margaret Ripple, who was attuned in 1998 by Wendy Koenig, who was attuned in 1997 by Laurie Allen Grant.

In 1989, Laurie Grant was attuned by James P. Davis, who was attuned by Dr. Arthur L. Robertson. Dr. Robertson was initiated in the 1970s into the Reiki system by Master teacher Virginia W. Samdahl, the first Occidental Reiki Master initiated by Hawayo Hiromi Takata.

In 1938, Mrs. Takata received her Master's attunement from Dr. Chujiro Hayashi. Dr. Hayashi is believed to be the last person who received his Reiki Mastership from Dr. Usui in 1925. And Dr. Usui received his attunement from Spirit on Mount Kurama in the early 1920s' from his findings in the ancient Sanskrit text.

Interesting Fact, Iris Ishikuro was one of Mrs. Takata's Master's students and was also her cousin. Iris also had other training, the Johrei Fellowship, a religion that includes healing with energy projected from the hands, another kind of Reiki from her sister who worked in a Tibetan temple in Hawaii, and another type of Reiki came to be called Raku Kei. Iris is the person known for changing Mrs. Takata's fee structure and who studied and shared her knowledge with Dr. Robertson.

How Reiki Energy Works

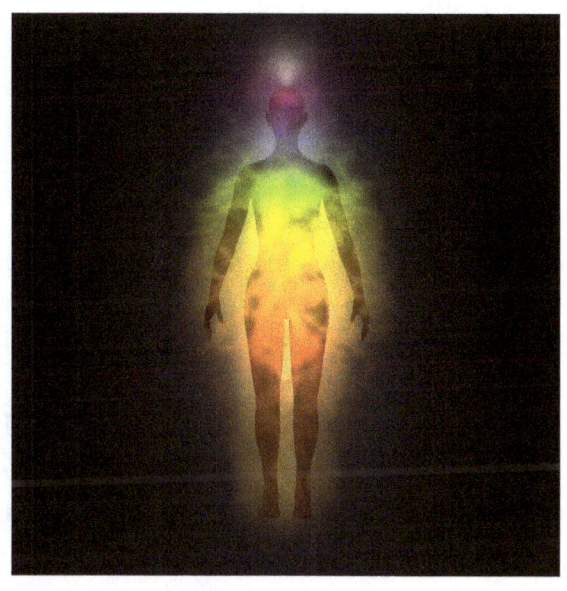

Reiki energy heals the person by flowing through the affected parts of the vital or auric field (aura) and balancing the area.

Each person has a field that surrounds their physical body. During a Reiki session, the cosmic energy raises the person's vibratory rate and frequency of their vital field (aura), balancing it.

Imagine, if you like, that the vital field (aura) is like a pool of water. The water can be polluted by adding toxins, such as chemicals, mud, or objects. The water can also become stale if it is not fed fresh oxygen or has any movement. And after time, green or blue algae can grow, and the water goes rancid, killing anything that enters.

Water is a known conductor; the clearer the water, the better its conductive ability. So even though your vital field (aura) is not liquid like water and is invisible to most people's naked eye, it radiates the clarity of your body, mind, and soul's pool of health.

During a Reiki session, the intent of the life-force energy coming down from the Cosmos is channeled through the person's crown, brow, throat, and heart chakra, then is channeled through their hands to the chakra and tsubu area(s) that need balancing.

When a person is attuned to 2nd and 3rd Degree Reiki, this energy heals and balances the emotional, mental, and spiritual bodies of the person as well as their physical body.

CONSTANCE'S REIKI INTERPRETATION

I love to use this simplified story to explain to my students what Reiki energy is and how it works.

Imagine a lamp in your home; it can be any size or color. All lamps have an electrical cord, a lamp fixture, and a light bulb to use the lamp properly.

Imagine you are the lamp fixture, the client or person you will work on is the light bulb, and God, Spirit, or your Reiki Master is the Ki (Chi) energy that flows through the electrical cord to light the bulb.

All you are is the facilitator, the lamp, the one needed to light the bulb. And without plugging in the lamp to an electrical socket in the wall, the light bulb would not come on.

I remember doing a science project in school where we had a potato and a small flashlight bulb. I found it amazing that a potato has enough energy to light the bulb for a moment. Now I, just like the potato, personally I do not have enough energy to heal my client. And if I try, I will burn out quickly. Only the Source has all the energy the client will ever need.

If you feel drained after a session, you gave your energy away, not the Cosmic energy granted through the Source.

Also, it is useless and a waste of energy to plug the electrical cord in without the bulb in the lamp. Ensure you always have a reason and the client's permission when doing a Reiki session. When your Reiki Master in Spirit comes to help you, do not waste their time.

The point is you are only the facilitator, not the energy itself. I have witnessed many miracles while practicing Reiki, but it is not me. It is only the energy from Spirit flowing through me.

FASCINATING FACT

Because you are vibrating at a higher frequency of energy, another thing that can happen while giving a Reiki session is that you may receive flashes of intuitive knowledge about yourself or the person you are treating (information about their condition or changes that would improve their health).

If this happens, inform the person of your insight(s), even if it does not feel appropriate or real. Then, it is up to the person to do something about the information and can choose to listen or not. It is their responsibility for their healing. *As the old saying goes, you can lead a horse to water, but you cannot make it drink.*

Nothing received intuitionally is too "weird" to be explored. It is important to remember when using the information on the Chakras that these references cannot replace the knowingness of your intuition.

An example, I had an eye accident when I was a year and a half old. Most people would never know that about me. It is almost impossible to see or notice it. Only during a Reiki session would one discover through their intuition that my eye problems were created by falling on an object or that as a child, I had a bicycle accident and saw the traumatic incident split seconds before it happened. These physical and emotional blocks could possibly hold an issue in my eye.

Sensing The Reiki Energy

Some people can sense energy, and others cannot.

Over the years of teaching, I have had hundreds of students learn the modality of Reiki. Unfortunately, not everyone can feel the energy (giving or receiving).

I remember this one class, particularly a combined Reiki Level I & II class, and I had five students. I had explained Reiki, and how it worked and had finished the attunement into Level II Reiki. The students were about to start learning how to heal others.

I had this one student who struggled to know when to move on to the next Chakra. She said she could not feel anything. The person she was working on said she thought she was receiving something. But no matter what, the student was becoming more and more stressed over not feeling something.

I stopped what we were doing and had all the students try to sense energy by sitting on a chair, and one by one, I blindfolded them. I had different students come up to them to see if they could sense anything. This particular student could not. I tried a few other things, but again nothing.

I finally prayed up and asked for help, the message I received back down was to teach her how to muscle test a yes and no answer, so I did the forward movement for yes, and a backward movement for no. It worked! She was able to muscle test if she was finished with the Chakra she was working on or not.

Whether you sense the energy or not, it does not mean it is not working. Most people cannot sense electricity moving through the walls of a room and through the cord of a lamp, but that does not mean that even though you have not turned the light bulb on, the energy is not working. I will not stick my finger into the socket to see if it is working.

After a time, you will know that the Reiki energy is working because of the miracles.

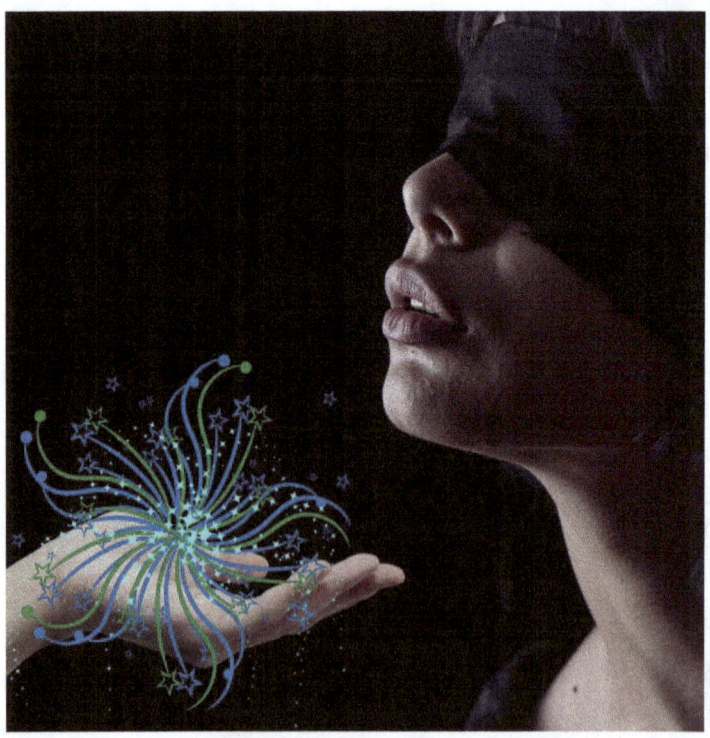

Basics of Level I Reiki

My gift to you is receiving 1st Degree (Level 1) Reiki for free. Everyone and their dog should know how to do Reiki (self-healing).

Go to my ConstanceSantego.ca website and follow Reiki Level I instructions.

All the Reiki techniques are based on these Seven Major Chakras:

- Crown
- Brow/Third eye
- Throat
- Heart
- Solar Plexus/Navel
- Sacral/ Spleen/Sexx
- Root/Base

For Self-Reiki, twenty-one minor Chakra hand positions (and the body's joints) exist.

- 1 – Crown Chakra
- 1 – Throat Chakra
- 2 – Shoulder
- 1 – Heart Chakra
- 2 – Crease of elbow
- 2 – Wrist of each hand
- 2 – Palm of each hand
- 1 – Solar Plexus Chakra
- 1 – Sacral Chakra
- 1 – Root Chakra
- 1 – Hips

- 2 – Behind each knee
- 2 – Ankle of each foot
- 2 – Sole of each foot

BUT, in Shiatsu, 361 Tsubo points run along the 12 meridians. *A Tsubo is any point along the surface of the body. Each meridian has a different number of points that you can activate, just like a Chakra.* You can hold any of these points during a Reiki session.

<u>Meridian</u>	<u>Points</u>
Lung	11 points
Large Intestine	20 points
Stomach	45 points
Spleen	21 points
Heart	9 points
Small Intestine	19 points
Bladder	67 points
(different charts number this meridian differently)	
Kidney	27 points
Pericardium or Circulation /Sex	9 points
Sanjiao or Triple Warmer	23 points
Gall Bladder	44 points
Liver	14 points
Ren Meridian or Conception Vessel/Central	24 points
Du Meridian or Governing Vessel/Governing	28 points

FREE GUIDE, go to
https://constancesantego.ca/education/workshops/reiki-level-1-courses/

SECRET OF A HEALER – MAGIC OF REIKI 107

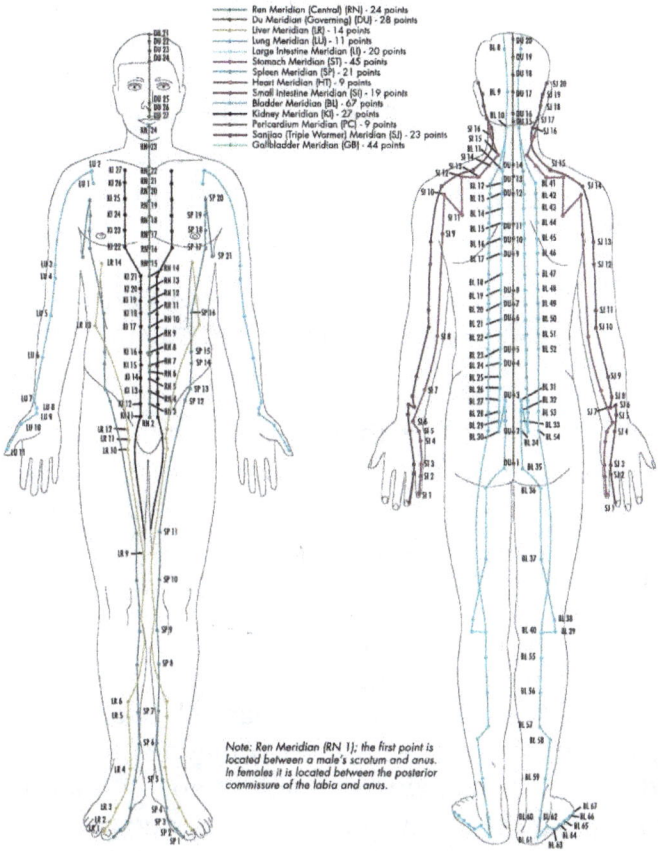

FIGURE 1: Anterior View of Meridians   FIGURE 2: Posterior View of Meridians

Note: Ren Meridian (RN 1); the first point is located between a male's scrotum and anus. In females it is located between the posterior commissure of the labia and anus.

***Meaning; these Tsubo are the points where energy can go into and out of the body—front and back. Each Tsubo can receive the Reiki energy to balance the meridian.

Reiki Master in Spirit

This is what sets apart Reiki's hand-on-healing compared to other modalities of hands-on-healing... You receive a Reiki Master in Spirit to help guide you during a Reiki session.

Everyone is granted a special companion (a type of Guiding Angel) whose job is to help you facilitate a Reiki session.

Your Reiki Master will be shown to you in your attunement to the Reiki energy. This is a very special experience; some people feel wonderful tingles, some see beautiful colors and images, some hear music, and some just know it to be true.

You will meet your Reiki Master through a meditation that I will read to you during the video presentation on my Constance Santego YouTube Channel. Everyone seems to receive as a Reiki Master someone or something a little different. It will always come to you in the form that you can handle. I have had students who get a person–male or female, old or young, some Jesus, some an Angel, some a Master, some an animal, some a mystical creature like a dragon, some a color, some just a name, and some are so scared they do not seem to get anything.

Just relax... and enjoy the meditation.

For the meditation, go to, https://www.youtube.com/watch?v=tdE4Kbod9r4&t=71s

Reiki Level I Attunement

You will need:

- Approximately 30 minutes
- Comfortable chair
- A small glass of lemon water

Reiki Attunement Procedure:

- Listen to the Reiki Level I video on my Constance Santego YouTube Channel.
- Get comfortable, but I suggest that you sit up. If you lie down, some students fall asleep. You may want to know what is going on around you.
- You will be guided through this wonderful meditation to clear yourself physically, emotionally, mentally, and spiritually.
- Partway through the meditation, I will ask you to do the Kidney Breath and Hui Yin while your Reiki Master opens your Chakras so you can later do Reiki.
- At the end of the meditation, I will ask you to do the Water Ritual while you read the Raku Kei Affirmation.

Kidney Breathing & The Hui Yin

When you are being attuned, during the meditation, I will direct the Raku fire energy up your spinal column and into your pineal gland. This re-energizes your entire body and raises your spiritual consciousness.

Place your hands over your kidneys (located on your lower back) for the kidney breath.

Your Hui Yin is an acupressure point between your anus and genitals (Root Chakra). Breathe normally while feeling like you are pulling this point into your body as you contract it.

As you take a breath, imagine the fire energy rising from your Root Chakra, up through your spine, entering and swirling in your head.

Place your tongue at the roof of your mouth behind your front teeth, and release this energy through your mouth.

Release your Hui Yin.

Water Ritual

Water purifies, conducts energy, and amplifies the effectiveness of the symbols one is attuned to.

Prepare the Water
- Get a small glass of water (2 oz)
- Pour ½ tsp of lemon juice into the glass
- Once you have the glass, your Reiki Master in Spirit will assist you in blessing the lemon water with the appropriate Reiki symbol.

Say the Raku Kei Affirmation and drink the lemon water, symbolizing cleansing your inside.

Raku Kei Affirmation

I believe there is a great cosmic magnet that manifests as the Spirit of truth, love, and light. This cosmic magnet lives in me as part of my divine nature.

I recognize the pure white light in my soul. This Holy Spirit in my soul continually guides me in everything I think, say, see, and do.

Through my magnetic personality, I pour my resources into the world. As I give, so shall I receive, living my life happily, expressing creatively, and experiencing perfect well-being.

So be it now and forever.

21-Day Cleanse

I suggest that you read my Angelic Lifestyle, A Vibrant Lifestyle Series.

Reiki is a powerful shift in energy. You may not notice the shift in your energy, but others around you will.

You may or may not sense a change in your body, mind, or soul. Some people's bodies do a physical purifying cleanse after receiving their attunement. It can be flu-like symptoms you may (or may not) feel.

As your body shifts in the frequency of this new energy, it may purge toxins. To lessen the effect, do self-Reiki treatments, talk long walks, deep breaths, drink lots of water, and eat light, nourishing meals.

You may also have an emotional, mental, or spiritual cleanse if you start to feel negative emotions, lovingly give them up and let them go. Place one hand on your forehead and the other on your belly button to lessen the effects. Visualize the beautiful white light coming into your crown Chakra, circulating throughout your body, or take an Epsom salt bath (1 cup Epsom salt). Or listen to the negative energy release Meditation on my Constance Santego YouTube Channel.

Not everyone feels a flu-like symptom. However, I felt no negative effects during or after my attunements.

PART THREE

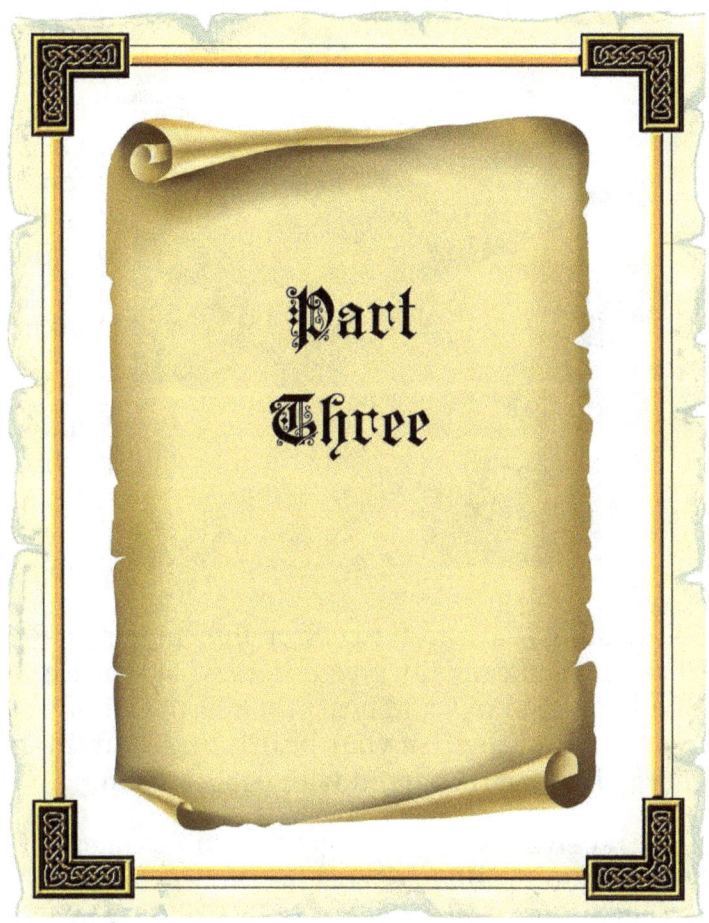

Reiki Self-Treatment

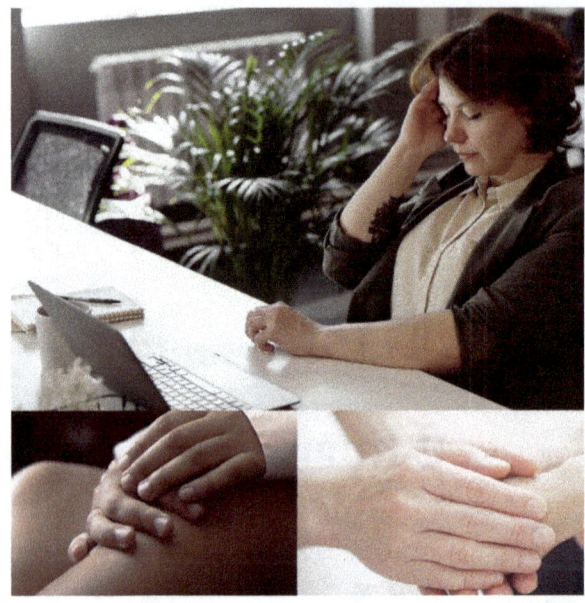

Self-healing, you do it naturally. Now do it with the intent of bringing down the life-force healing energy used in Reiki.

You can do Reiki while reading, listening to music, or watching TV.

Self-healing is a crucial first step in becoming a Reiki Channel. You can only give others what you are willing to give yourself. Love and heal yourself first! Daily self-treatments strengthen your health, and your life-force energy is being recharged with each session.

After receiving your 1st Degree Reiki Attunement, your energy system will have to adjust to the higher vibration. However, this energy will balance itself out in a noticeably short time.

Procedure

1. Make yourself comfortable by sitting or lying down.

2. Call upon your Reiki Master in Spirit and your higher self to assist you in this treatment. If you are attuned to 2nd or 3rd Degree Reiki, use the symbols.
3. Close your eyes and pay attention to the rhythm of your breathing.
4. Rub your hands together.
5. Place one hand on your Solar Plexus (Navel) Chakra.
6. Place your other hand on your Sacral (Spleen/Sexx) Chakra.
7. Intent or ask that the Reiki energy flows through you at the highest level that is beneficial for you.
8. Follow the twenty-one minor hand positions as directed until you intuitively sense where to place your hands.

Go to my Constance Santego WEBSITE for the FREE Reiki hand position guidebook (under Level I Reiki).

Front and Back Positions for the Body
1. Head/Crown & Brow Chakra – 5 positions
2. Neck/Throat Chakra – 2 positions
3. Shoulders – 2 positions
4. Heart/Heart Chakra – 2 positions
5. Ribcage/Solar Plexus Chakra – 1 position
6. Bellybutton/ Sacral Chakra – 1 position
7. Groin/Root Chakra – 1 position
8. Back – 3 positions
9. Elbows – 2 positions
10. Wrists and Hands – 4 positions
11. Knee, Ankle & Feet – 6 positions

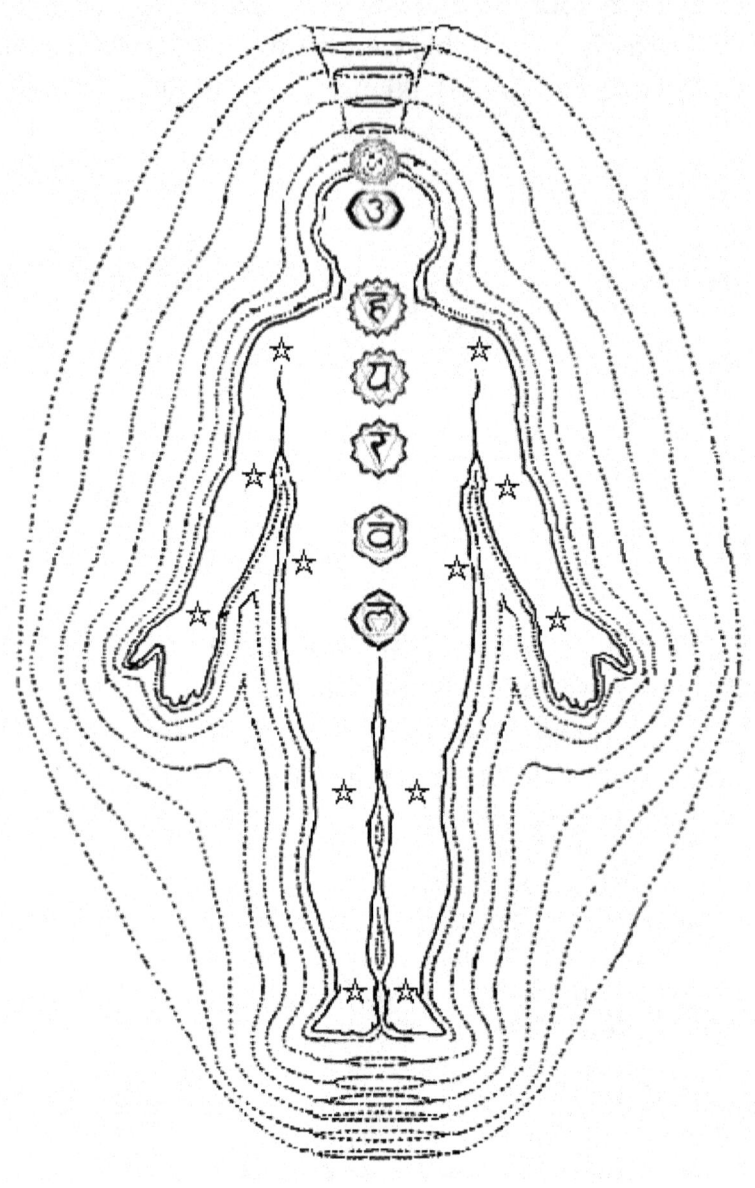

A Reiki Mantra

After a self-healing session, say, 'I ask that this Reiki energy continue to heal, harmonize, and balance my top with my bottom, my front with my back, my inside with my outside, my left with my right, and my yin with my yang. I also ask that this Reiki energy continue to heal, harmonize, and balance my body, mind, spirit, and emotions.'

Or just thank your Reiki Master in Spirit for helping me.

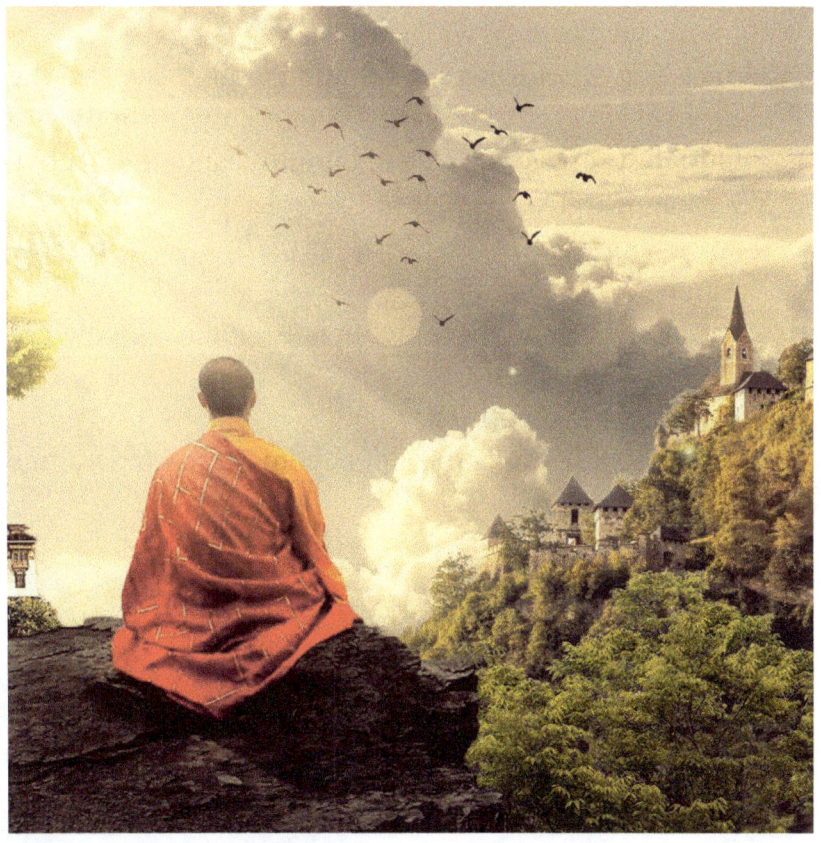

Reiki Breathing Exercise

1. Make yourself comfortable by sitting or lying down.
2. Call upon your Reiki Master in Spirit
3. Close your eyes and pay attention to the rhythm of your breathing.
4. Rub your hands together.
5. Intuitively, place your hands on two of your Chakras (any two).
6. Now imagine the life-force energy and consciously direct your breath through your hands and into the Chakras you hold.
7. Notice any feelings of relaxation and peace as the sensation gradually spreads throughout your body.
8. Hold these areas for a few minutes, and then move your hands to two new Chakras.
9. Allow yourself to let go of any rhyme or reason. Breathe.
10. Continue the hand placements until you have covered all seven Chakras at least once.
11. Focus on your breathing.
12. When you are finished, open your eyes, and notice how you feel now.

Reiki Quick Energizer

1. Make yourself comfortable by sitting or lying down.
2. Call upon your Reiki Master in Spirit
3. Rub your hands together.
4. Place one hand on your Solar Plexus (Navel) Chakra.
5. Place your other hand directly under it, touching your stomach.
6. Close your eyes, relax your hands, and let your mind drift.
7. Hold that position for 5 to 15 minutes.
8. When you are finished, open your eyes, and notice how rejuvenated and refreshed you feel.

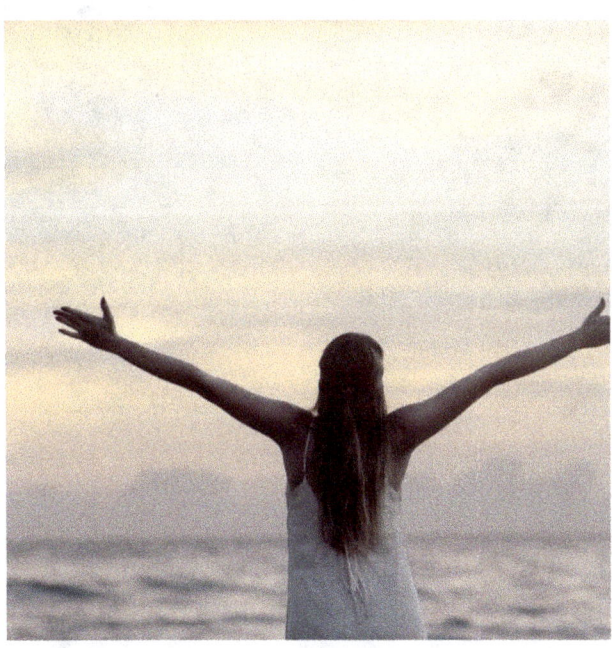

Reiki For Your Electronics

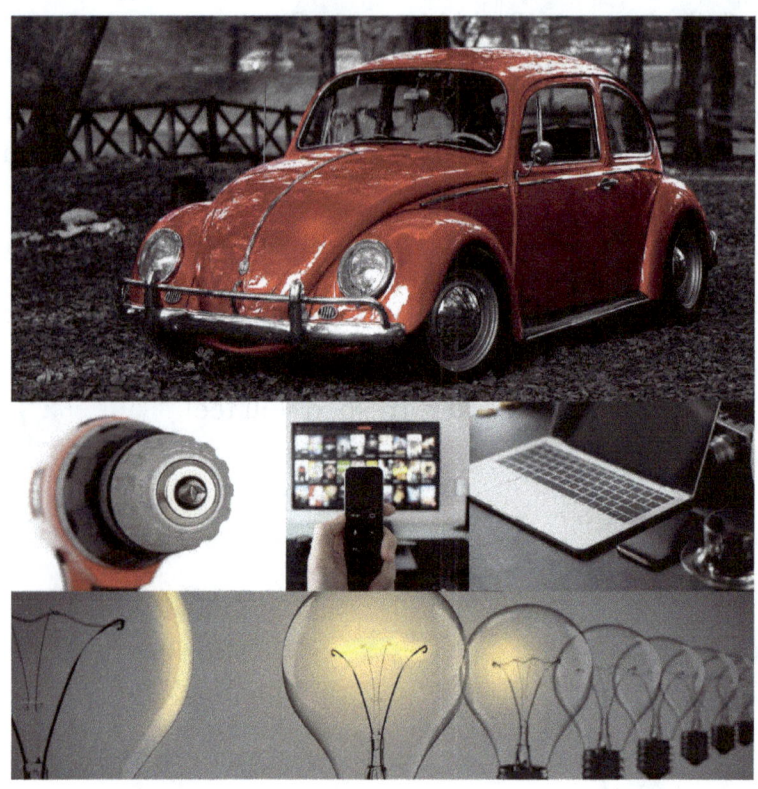

𝔐y husband is exceptionally good at this. He has used the Reiki technique to fix many electronics when they have gone on the fritz. Like a friend's car when the battery died, my till at work, computers, and his tools.

Give it a try. You might impress yourself.

Reiki For Your Pets

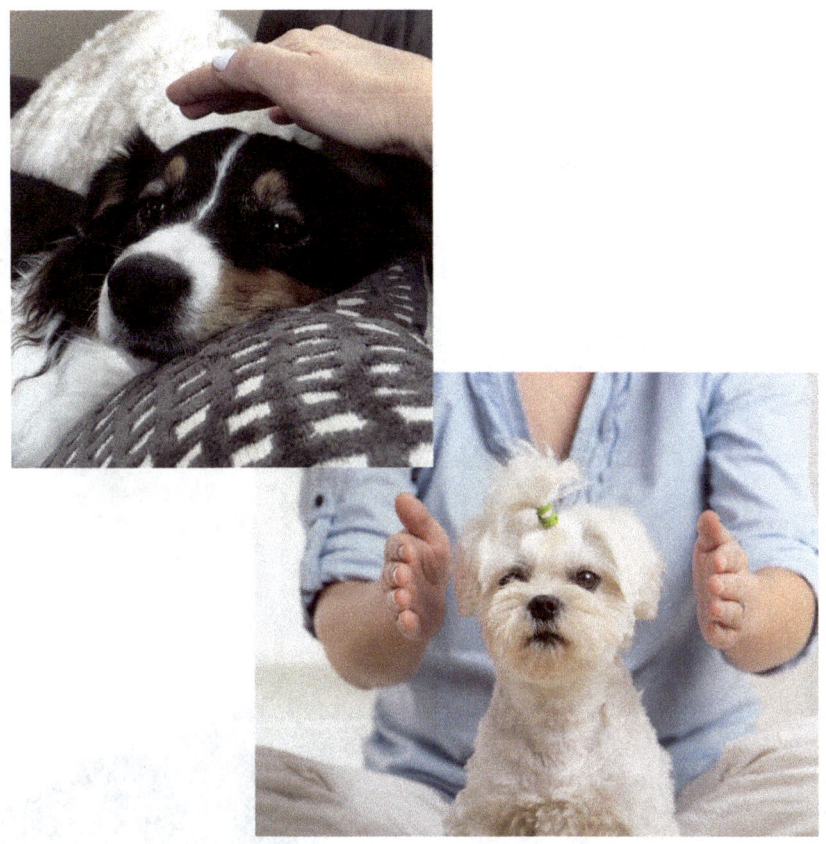

Most animals will love receiving a Reiki session.

Reiki For Your Plants

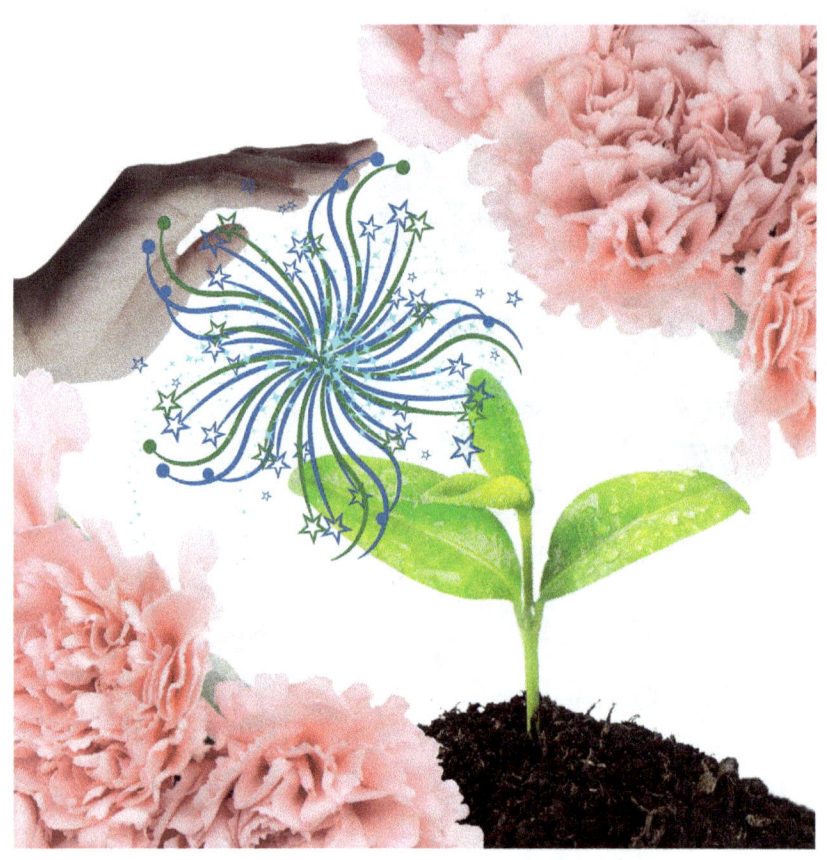

Use Reiki energy to help your plants grow.

Reiki For Sleep

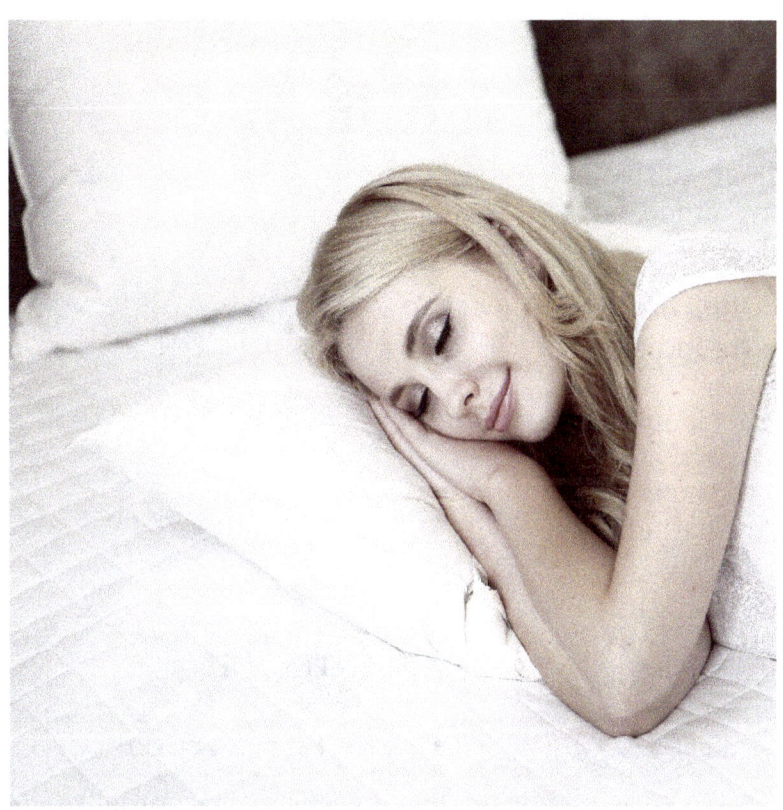

1. Lie down and make yourself comfortable.
2. Call upon your Reiki Master in Spirit
3. Rub your hands together.
4. Place one hand on your Sacral (Spleen/Sexx) Chakra.
5. Place your other hand on your Brow Chakra.
6. Notice your breath going in and out.
7. Remain in that position until the Reiki energy generates a feeling of deep relaxation.

Aromatherapy For Chakras

Essential Oils have been used for centuries to cure ailments of the body, mind, and soul.

For full detail of contra-indications and how to blend, check out my Secrets of a Healer – Magic of Aromatherapy Book.

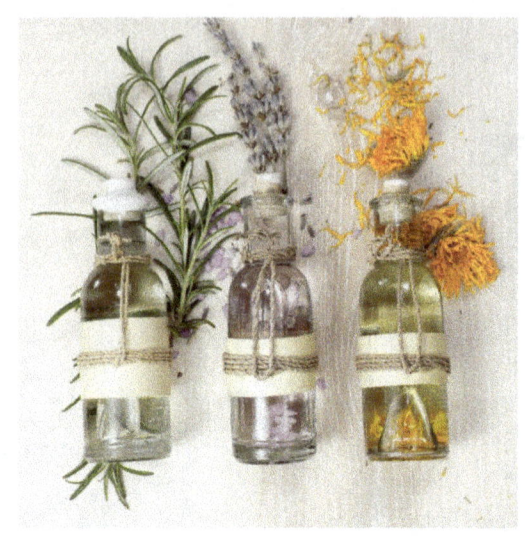

CHAKRA	ESSENTIAL OIL
Root	Cedar, Clove, Pepper, Vetiver
Sacral	Melissa, Orange Oil, Damiana, Gardenia, Sandalwood, Ylang-Ylang
Solar Plexus	Rosemary, fennel, bergamot, grapefruit, lemon, lemongrass, petitgrain, marigold
Heart	Eucalyptus, Pine Oil, Marjoram, Orrisroot, Rose Oil, Yarrow
Throat	Geranium, Chamomile Oil, Benzoin, Eucalyptus, Frankincense, Sage
Brow	Jasmine, Mint, Mugwort, Star Anise
Crown	Lotus, Rose, Spruce

Chakra Stone Technique

Make the client comfortable lying down face up on a table. *They will keep their clothes on.*

Cover the client with a blanket. Center and ground yourself.

Step 1) Put **one warm stone in each hand of the client**. Say out loud to the client...

> "**With the stones' warmth, go inside yourself and notice your breathing... Relax... Let go... Knowing that you are safe... Make yourself comfortable... Go inside and release any negative thoughts... Imagine beautiful light color and bring it in .... Relax and let go... Enjoy...**"

Step 2) Start the session by putting an **aroma blend on your hands, and then hover over the client's face** while they take in three deep breaths.

Step 3) Get one **small warm stone** *(make sure it is dry)* **and rub in small slow circles on each Chakra. Leave** the stone on the charka. Repeat with each charka: Crown Chakra *(top of head)* Brow *(between eyebrows)* Throat *(very lightly on throat* Heart *(high heart above breast area, and a little to the left)* Solar plexus *(center of the body and under the ribcage)* Spleen *(above belly button)* Root *(choose one side and do closer to hip)*

> While waiting, do a **light massage of the hands** (can use cream), then do a light **foot** rub through their socks.

Step 4) Go up the chakras, starting at Root Chakra and going to the Crown. **Lightly finger tap the stone** of each

Chakra **while very quietly saying all the Mental/Emotional sentences** first and then all positive words in that Chakra. Then do the next Chakra...

Chakra Mental, Emotional Positive Words

1. Root Physical family, group safety, security, Relaxation, Ability to provide for life's necessities, Peace, Social and familiar law and order, Tranquility, Ability to stand up for self, Generosity, Feeling at home, Confidence, Inner Direction, Calmness, Assurance

2. Spleen Blame and guilt, Self-belief, Money and Sex, Consideration, Power and control, Understanding, Creativity, Joyfulness, Ethics, and honor in relationships, Nourishing, Self-worth, Enthusiasm, Compassion, Contentment

3. Solar Plexus Trust, Harmony, Fear and intimidation, Love, Self-esteem, self-confidence, self-respect, Adoration, Care of oneself and others, Motivation, Responsibility for making decisions, Humbleness, Sensitivity to criticism, Choice, Personal honor, Pride, Transformation, Responsibility, Forgiveness

4. Heart Love and hatred, Empathy, Resentment and bitterness, Self-confidence, Grief and anger, Self-respect, Self-centeredness, Confidence, Loneliness, commitment, Love, Forgiveness and compassion, Cheerfulness, Hope and trust, Humbleness, Modesty, Sincerity,

5. Throat Choice and strength of will, Lightness, Personal expression, Balance, following one's dream, Buoyancy, using personal power to create, Addiction, Judgment and criticism, Faith and knowledge, Capacity to make decisions

6. Brow Self-evaluation, Success, Truth, Self-Respect, Intellectual abilities, Feelings of adequacy, openness to the ideas of others, Ability to learn from experience, Emotional intelligence

7: Crown Ability to trust life, Honesty, Values, Ethics, Courage Trust, Humanitarianism, Truth, Selflessness, Ability to see the larger pattern, Faith and inspiration, Spirituality, and devotion

Step 5) Once you have done all the Chakras, **lightly tap two stones** over each Chakra while **humming the 'OM' sound**. The light tapping of the two basalt stones sends negative ions out. *(A very good thing in healing)*

Step 6) End the session by putting the **aroma blend** on your hands and **hovering over the client's face** while they take three deep breaths.

Crystal Chakra Release

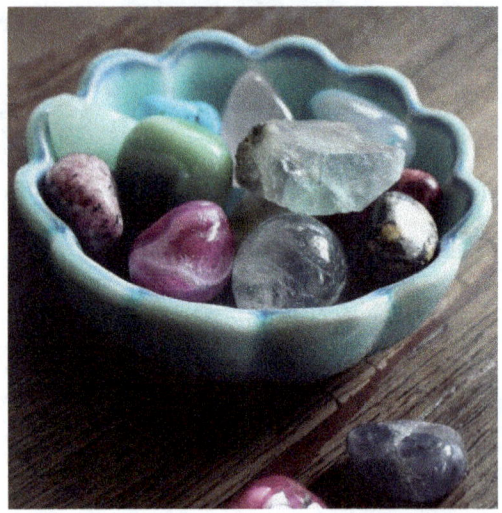

1. You will need a scale and nine stones (any color, any type).
2. Weigh all the stones individually and write them down. Put the stones into a cup.
3. Have a friend lie down. You may put a blanket on them (ensure they are comfortable).
4. Place a stone on each of the Chakras, one at the top of their head and the bottom of their feet.
5. Have them lie there for about ten to twenty minutes. If you know Reiki or similar, you may do that now.
6. When you are completed, remove the stones and place them back into the cup. Ask your client to take a few moments, and when ready, get up.
7. Reweigh the stones and write them down.
8. Clean the stones in water, sunlight/moonlight, or snow, and place them in a large crystal. However you like.
9. Reweigh the stones. Every person is different. The stones weigh less when the person needs/takes some energy. The stones weighed more when the person let go of some energy and the stone took it on.

Watch my Constance Santego YouTube Channel – Experiment #2 Energy . . .

Muscle Testing Chakra *for* Meditation

For the full details on Muscle Testing, read my book, "Secrets of a Healer – Magic of Muscle Testing." to watch a Muscle Testing demo, go to my Constance Santego YouTube Channel.

Procedure: 1st Muscle Test the Chakra that is off and needs balancing.

1. Root
2. Sacral
3. Solar Plexus
4. Heart
5. Throat
6. Brow
7. Crown

2nd Hold the appropriate Reiki hand positions during the meditation.

3rd, Either have someone read you the meditation in this book or go to my Constance Santego YouTube Channel and listen to that specific Chakra meditation.
Extras:

- o Have a Chakra-colored bath while listening to the meditation.
- o Hold the appropriate crystal while doing the meditation.
- o Light a candle that is the appropriate Chakra color.
- o Burn the appropriate incense for that Chakra.
- o Use the appropriate aromatherapy for that Chakra (in the bath or on a tissue).

Negative Energy & Chakra Clearing Meditation

1. Make yourself comfortable in a chair or lie down
2. When you are ready, close your eyes.
3. Imagine your *Root Chakra* (the lowest point of your torso)
    a. Imagine a <u>red</u> flower opening… any type of flower will do,

    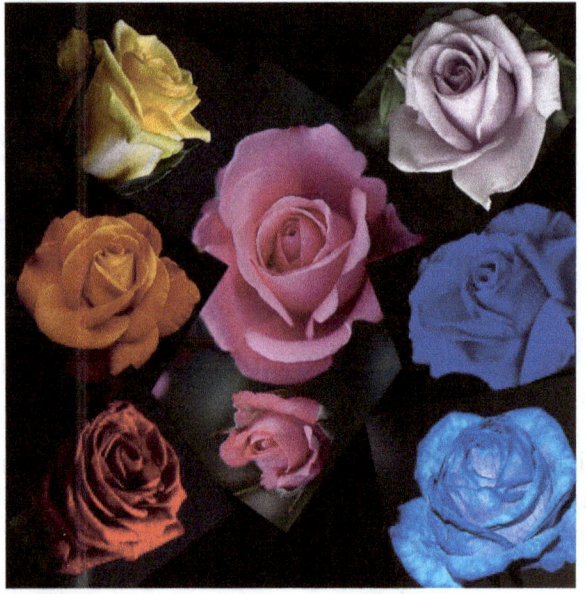

    b. Imagine that there are cords attached to you here. The Huna or Kundalini called these 'aka' cords.
    c. Now imagine all of these cords that are not yours being released lovingly to whomever they belong to and all of yours returning to you.

d. You can imagine releasing them like you would a cable from your computer or phone,
   e. Great, now wait a few moments while this Chakra is being cleansed
   f. If there are too many to release right now, know that you can always come back to this Chakra again later,
   g. Take a deep breath,
   h. Imagine a clear bubble forming over the top of this area for protection.
4. Imagine your *Sacral or Sex Chakra* (the area between your root and belly button).
   a. Imagine an <u>orange</u> flower opening...
   b. Imagine these aka cords that are attached to you here,
   c. Again, imagine all of these cords that are not yours being released lovingly to whomever they belong to and all of yours coming back to you,
   d. And wait again a few moments while this Chakra is being cleansed,
   e. Take a deep breath,
   f. Imagine a clear bubble over the top of this area for protection.
5. Now, imagine your *Solar Plexus or Navel Chakra* (from belly button to bottom of sternum)
   a. Imagine a <u>yellow</u> flower opening...
   b. Imagine lovingly releasing all the aka cords back to whomever they belong to and all of yours returning to you.
   c. Excellent, now wait again a few moments while this next Chakra is being cleansed.

d. Know that if there are too many to release right now and you can always come back to this Chakra again later,
e. Take a deep breath,
f. Imagine a clear bubble over the top of this area for protection.
6. Imagine your *Heart Chakra* (between the solar plexus and your throat)
    a. Imagine a <u>green</u> or pink flower opening…
    b. Imagine the aka cords being released lovingly to whomever they belong to and all of yours returning to you.
    c. Wait again a few moments while this Chakra is being cleansed,
    d. Take a deep breath,
    e. Imagine a clear bubble over the top of this area for protection.
7. Imagine your *Throat Chakra* (all your neck area)
    a. Imagine a <u>blue</u> flower opening…
    b. Imagine the aka being released lovingly to whomever they belong to and all of yours coming back to you.
    c. Wait again while this Chakra is being cleansed,
    d. Take a deep breath,
    e. Imagine a clear bubble over the top of this area for protection.
8. Imagine your *Brow or Third eye Chakra* (your forehead area)
    a. Imagine an <u>indigo</u> flower opening up…(a purple/blue color like cobalt blue)
    b. Imagine all these cords being released lovingly to whomever they belong to and all of yours returning to you.

c. Take a moment while this Chakra is being cleansed,
   d. Take a deep breath,
   e. Imagine a clear bubble over the top of this area for protection.
9. Imagine your *Crown Chakra* (top of your head, the baby's soft spot)
   a. Imagine a <u>violet</u> flower opening...
   b. Imagine all these cords being released lovingly to whomever they belong to and all of yours returning to you.
   c. Wait for this Chakra to be cleansed,
   d. Again, if there are too many to release right now and you can always come back to this Chakra again later,
   e. Take a deep breath,
   f. Imagine a clear bubble over the top of this area for protection.
10. Perfect, now that you have cleansed the main Chakras, I want you to imagine,
    a. Beautiful crystal-clear light energy coming down from the heavens and entering your crown Chakra,
    b. Let this light flow down your spinal column and up through the root Chakra right up through to the crown Chakra,
    c. This light flows out of the crown Chakra like a water fountain and into your aura,
    d. Imagine you have an aura about three feet extended from you in all positions; above, behind, to the sides, and below you.
    e. Bringing this beautiful crystal-clear light energy down from the heavens that continually

cleanses all your Chakras and flows into your aura to cleanse it.
   f. Now, as this beautiful energy comes into your aura, think positive words or affirmations,
   g. Imagine these positive words vibrating in your cleansed aura,
   h. Manifesting your dreams, wishes, wants, and desires into reality.
11. Marvelous, now take a deep breath and imagine this cleansed energy being sealed into your body and aura.
12. Take another deep breath, wiggle your toes, and open your eyes, returning to the moment.
13. Feeling wonderfully rejuvenated and energized!

Pendulum Chakra Release

1. You will need a pendulum. This can be a charm on a necklace, a small Christmas ball on a string, or anything that swings.
2. Have a friend lie down. You may put a blanket on them (ensure they are comfortable).
3. Start at any Chakra, including the feet.
4. Hold the pendulum above the person, not having it touch them. Say to yourself, *"Pendulum move in any direction needed to clear this Chakra."* Wait until it starts to move, and then wait until it stops. You may change hands if you get tired. This may take a moment, or it may take many. Sometimes if the pendulum is going forever, ask the person to take a breath and wiggle their toes.
5. Complete this on all the Chakras.
6. When finished, take a breath, and give thanks.

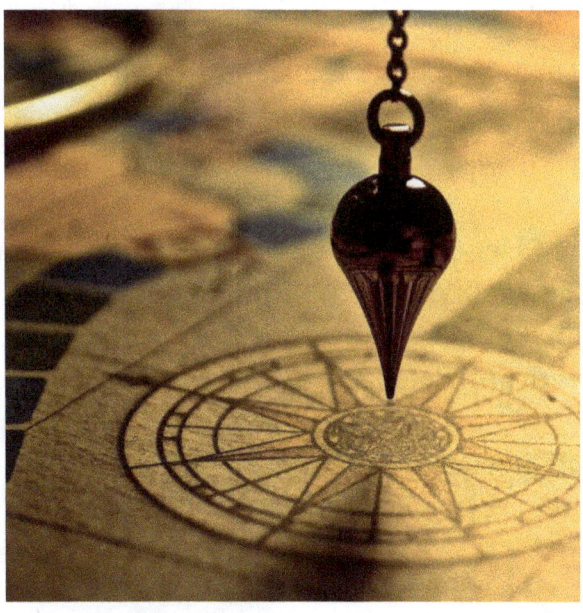

Sound Essence Chakra Balancers

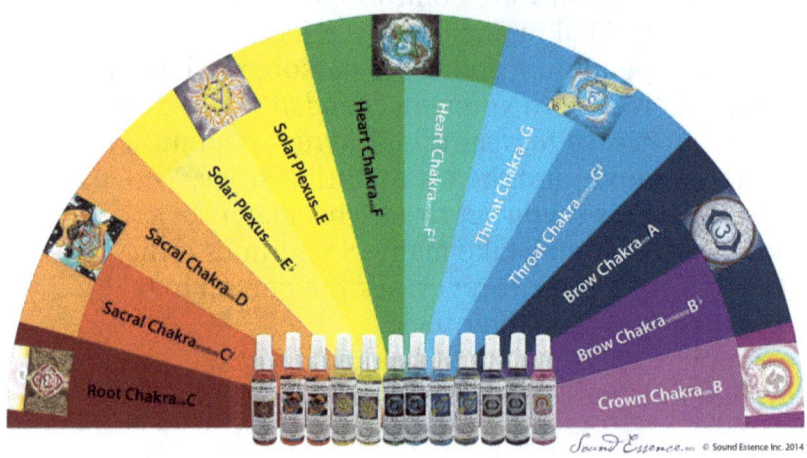

Chakra Balancer Sound Essence™ are subtle energy remedies created from the healing vibration of sound from crystal bowls.

Each Sound Essence™ holds vibrational information that supports the vitality of the human energy system. These information therapies resonate at various frequencies and interface with any field lacking vibration.

Vibrational information is as vital to our energy system as air and water are to our physical system.

What Makes Them Special
The Chakra Balancer Sound Essence™
- Hold the imprint of the vibration of each whole note *and* semitone of the harmonic scale,
    - sound
- Have the equivalent color of the chromatic scale,
    - color
- And are jointly charged with the information imprint of chosen:
    - crystals and gemstones,
    - sacred geometry,
    - ancient symbology,
    - positive word vibrations,
    - aromatherapy.

The whole notes resonate with the seven main chakras. The five semitones are bridges for the seven chakras (located on the back of the body, supporting the transitional aspects of the spine).

How To Use The Chakra Balancer Sound Essence™
These remedies are so simple to use.
Choice #1 – Use your intuition and choose your essence.
Choice #2 – If you know which Chakra needs balancing, use the appropriate essence.
Then - Lightly shake the bottle, close your eyes, simply mist the Chakra Balancer Sound Essence™ above and in front of yourself, and then step under the falling mist.

Shift Your Frequency!
Symphony of Vibration in a Bottle.
www.soundessence.net

Tuning Forks Chakra Balance

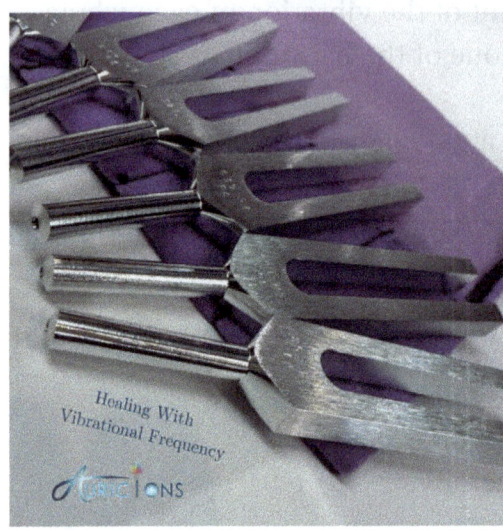

There are tuning forks that touch your body (weighted) and ones that hover over your body (unweighted).

For Spiritual Healing -Energy, Chakra, or Aura

- 1088.8Hz – Grounding & Balancing
- 544.4 Hz – Creating
- 272.2 Hz – Tissue Healing
- 544.4 + 272.2 = 816.6 Hz – Emotional Coding

For Physical Healing

- 201.42 Hz – Tissue healing
- 105.21 Hz – Muscle

For Spiritual & Mental Healing - Mix

- 1088.8 – 105.21 = 983.59 Hz – Imagery
- 544.4 – 105.21 = 429.19 Hz – Thinking

Tuning Fork Therapy uses sound vibration. Because our human bodies are not solid but rhythmic and harmonic, tuning forks can assist the immune system and help stimulate the body to heal itself.

The body is an awesome resonator for sound because sound resonates four times faster in water. These vibratory sounds travel through the body to help remove energetic blockages, relieving stasis and pain and increasing the flow of chi.

Using Tuning Forks on the body is a delightful and effective healing method that can be used on acupressure points, trigger and reflex points, bone, muscle, and tendons to help relieve pain or tonify and attune the body on a cellular level.

You can purchase individual Chakra Tuning Forks

CHAKRA	COLOR	NOTE	HZ FREQUENCY
Root	Red	C	256 Hz
Sacral	Orange	D	288 Hz
Solar Plexus	Yellow	E	320 Hz
Heart	Green	F	341.3 Hz
Throat	Blue	G	384 Hz
Brow	Indigo	A	426.7 Hz
Crown	Violet	B	480 Hz
Higher octave of Root	Red	C	512 Hz

www.energyvibration.com chart

BONUS - Healing Pool

This is a different type of energy healing.

Procedure:

1. Relax by taking three deep breaths.
2. Imagine you are walking on a pathway that leads to a building...
3. You will enter the building and go to the backdoor...
4. You will go out through the backdoor and enter a garden... This garden has a healing pool with a flowing waterfall.
    a. The water is a perfect temperature...
    b. This water is magical and will heal anything that enters it...
5. Go ahead and enter the water...
    a. Clothed, naked, swimsuit – you decide what you are wearing
    b. You can even breathe underwater.
    c. Your body can become completely buoyant if you want to float. There is no way of drowning.
    d. If you would rather, you may sit at the edge and have your feet or hands touch the water...
6. You may stay as long as you like.
    a. This may be a few moments,
    b. hours,
    c. days
    d. or years.

When I do this for a client, I bring them to the pool and make sure they are comfortable, and then I tell them that they can stay as long as they like and that I am leaving but will check in on them from time to time.

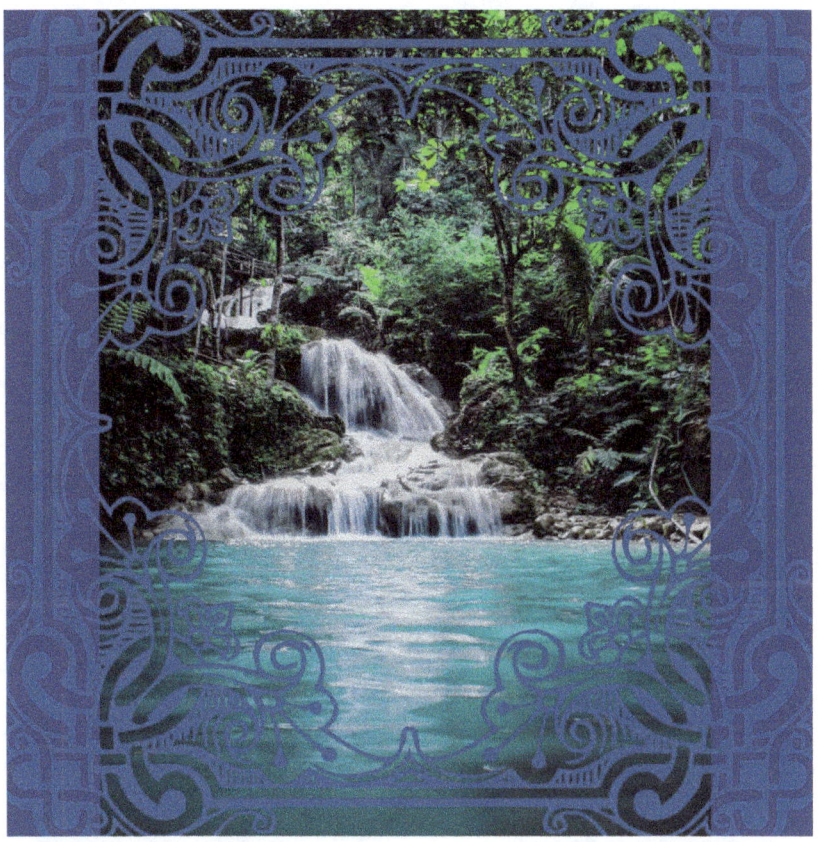

I must tell you an interesting story that happened to me many years ago. I had imagined bringing a lady into a healing pool.

When I imagined that we got there, pointing, she yelled, "I'm not getting into that pool with him!" Startled by her reaching into MY dream, I looked to where she was pointing, and a man was in the pool. I had forgotten days before I had brought another client to the pool.

Praying up, I asked, *"What do I do?"*

The answer was, *"Bring her to her own healing pool."*

So, I did.

Later I asked up again to find out how many healing pools there were. The answer was more of a picture, it was as if a waterfall backdrop scenery curtain fell to the ground revealing thousands of pools, and then the curtain was brought back into place again.

I never made the mistake of bringing a person to an occupied pool again.

Okay, maybe it is only me, but it did shock me. It was my dream. Why did my mind create the lady to yell? All I know is that the pool works. Many, many clients have told me of their miraculous healings.

Charts

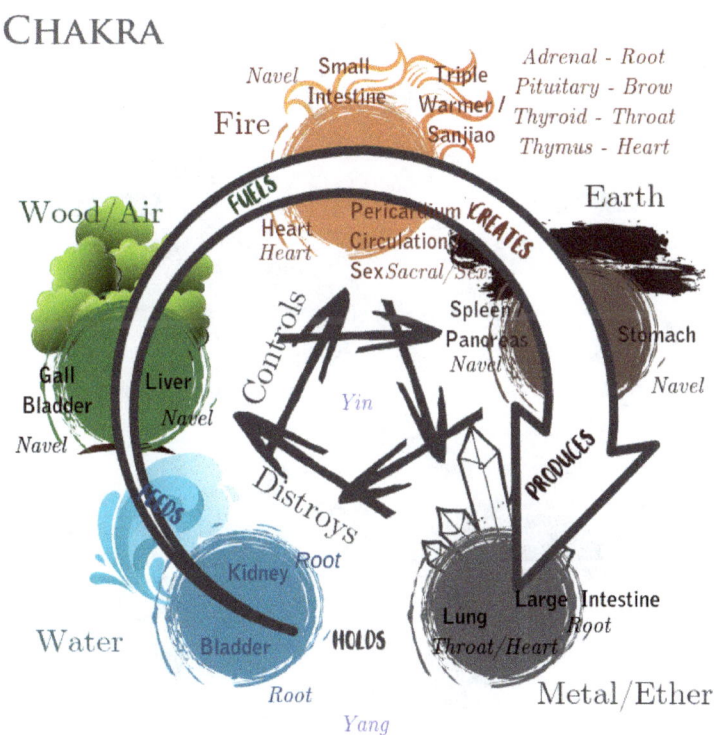

Energy

Crown
Bliss
God Consciousness
Upward Intuition

Brow
Supra-Mental
Human Intuition

Throat
Mental
Communication

Heart
Vital
Love

Solar Plexus/Navel
Vital
Will Power

Sacral/Sex
Physical
Family, Friends, Community

Root
Physical
All About You

BASIC ENERGY

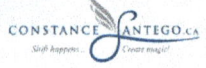

Feelings

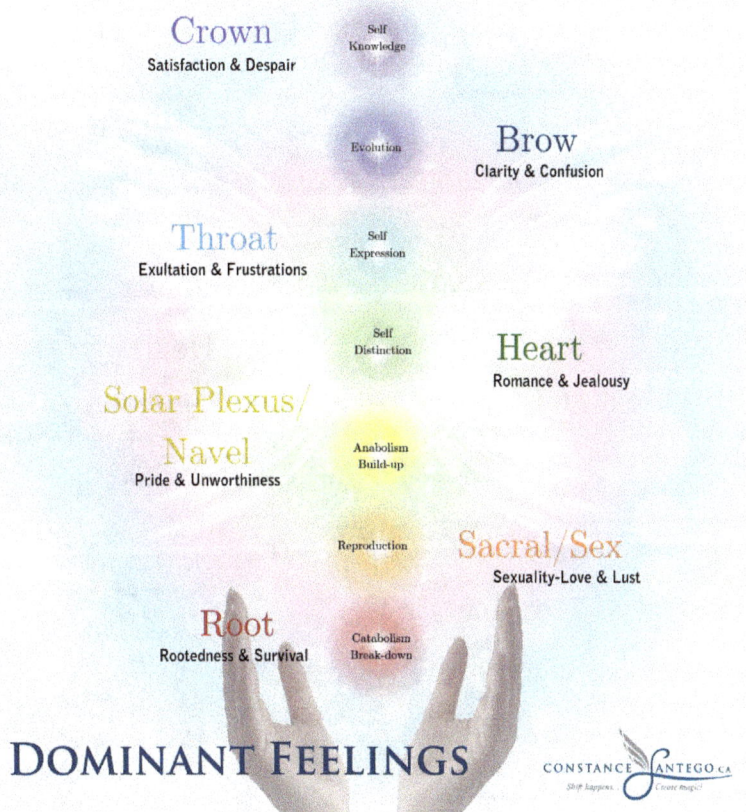

Dominant Feelings

Meridians

Crown
Pineal
Neocortex

Brow
Pituitary
Hindbrain
Midbrain
Eyes

Throat
Thyroid
Lung (voice)
Throat
Speech Organs

Heart
Heart
Lung (Chen)
Thymus

Solar Plexus/Navel
Small Intestine
Stomach
Spleen / Pancreas
Liver
Gall Bladder

Sacral/Sex
Pericardium / Cir/ Sex
- Prostrate
- Uterus
- Testies/Ovaries
Kidney (L)

Root
Adrenal
Kidney (R)
Bladder
Large Intestine/ Anus/ Rectum

5 Element

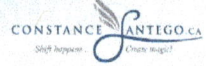

Musical Notes

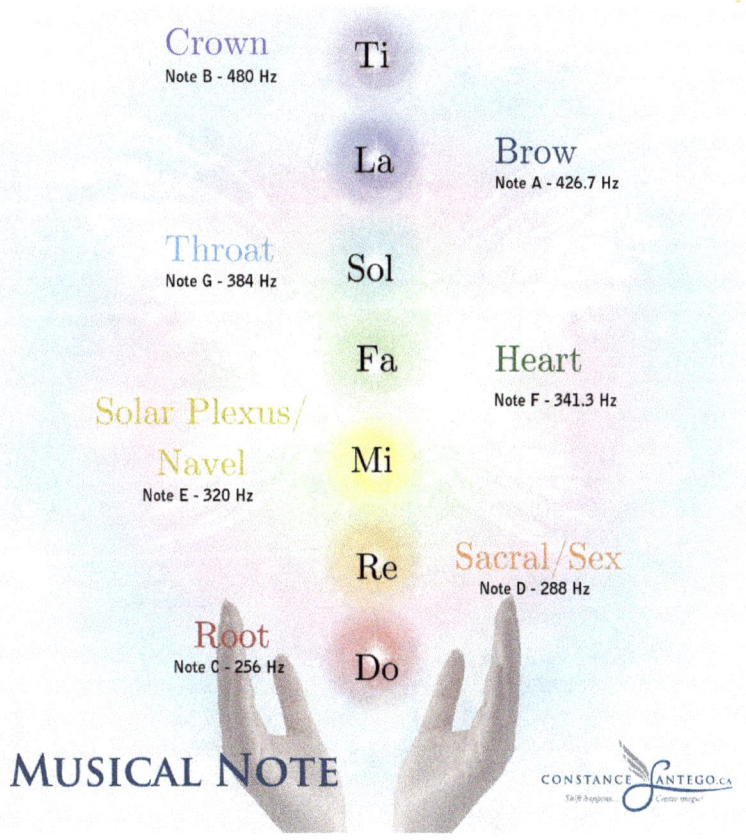

Organs & Glands

Crown
Central Nervous System, Pineal

Brow
Autonomic Nervous System, Pituitary, Pineal

Throat
Thyroids

Heart
Heart, Thymus

Solar Plexus/ Navel
Stomach, Spleen, Pancreas, Liver, Gall Bladder, Small Intestines

Sacral/Sex
Sex, Reproductive Organs

Root
Elimination Organs: Large Intestines, Kidney, Bladder, Adrenals

Organs & Glands

CONSTANCE SANTEGO.CA

Senses

Crown
Thought
Affirmations, Intent, Goals

Ti

La

Brow
Color & Light
Aura, Chakra

Throat
Sound
Music & Positive Words

Sol

Fa

Heart
Touch
Massage, Reflexology

Solar Plexus/
Navel
Sight
Imagery, Dreams

Mi

Re

Sacral/Sex
Taste
Food, Herbs

Root
Smell
Aromatherapy, Fragrances

Do

TO BALANCE

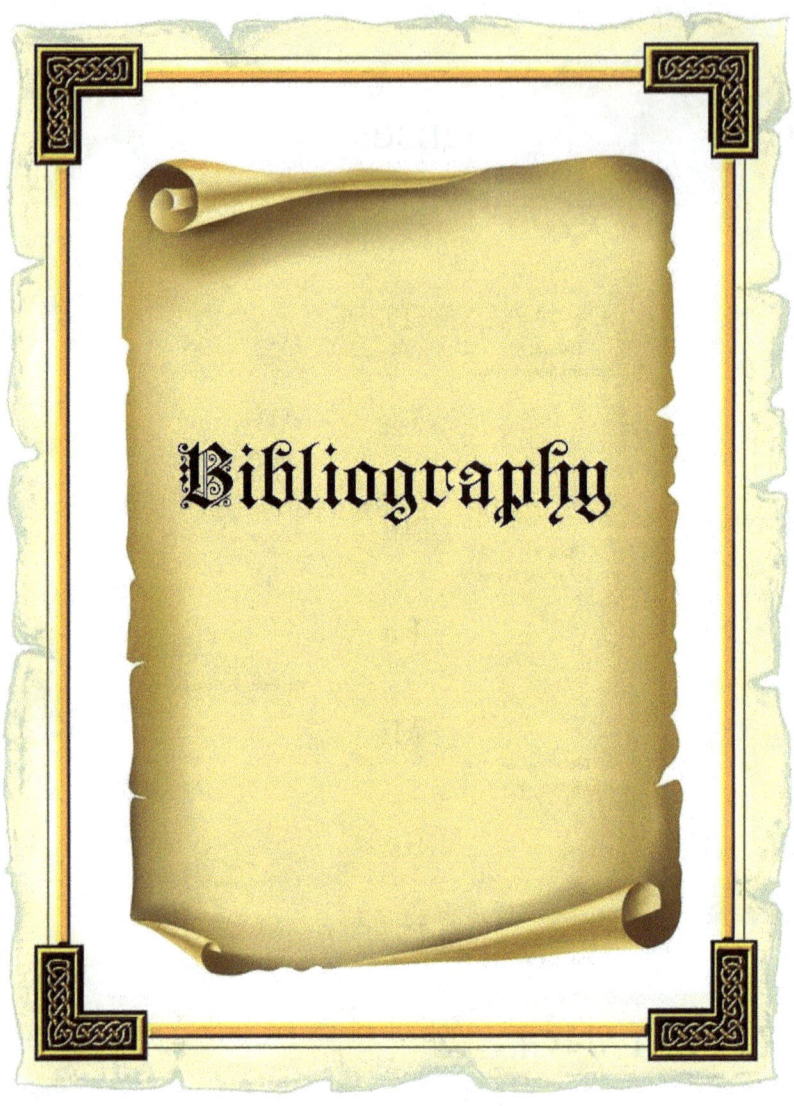

Bibliography

Much of this information was taken from the course information created when I owned the Canadian Institute of Natural Health and Healing Accredited College

Quantum University www.quantumuniversity.com

Artwork – www.canva.com

Associations
https://iarp.org/history-of-Reiki/

A Suggested Reading List

There are many books available to further your learning on the topics covered in this course; those listed here are some suggestions:

Ascended Masters

King, Godfrey Ray

          Unveiled Mysteries (Saint Germain Series; Vol.1).

    1989   The Magic Presence (Saint Germain Series; Vol. 2).

Sandweiss, Samuel H.

>1975   Sai Baba: The Holy Man and the Psychiatrist. San Diego, California: Birth Day Publishing Company

Stone, Joshua David

>1995   Ascended Masters Light the Way. Sedona, Arizona: Light Technology. Publications.

Aura and Psychometry

Brennan, Barbara

>1988   Hands of Light: a Guide to Healing Through the Human Energy Field. Bantam Books.

Chakras

Arguelles, Jose

>1987   The Mayan Factor: Path Beyond Technology.

Beinfield, Harriet and Korngold, Efrem

>1991   A Guide to Chinese Medicine. New York: Ballantine Books.

Castaneda, Carlos

>1974   Tales of Power. New York, New York: Pocket Books

Energy Healing

Brennan, Barbara Ann

    1987   Hands of Light. New York, New York: Bantam Books.

Guides

Altea, Rosemary

    1995   The Eagle and the Rose. New York, New York: Warner Books Inc.

Eadie, Betty J.

    1992   Embraced By The Light. New York: Bantam Books.

    1996   The Awakening Heart. New York, New York: Pocket Books.

Guggenheim, Bill

    1995   Hello From Heaven. New York: Bantam Books.

Van Praagh, James

    1997   Talking to Heaven. New York, New York: Penguin Group

Healing

Steiger, Brad

> 1971   Kahuna Magic. Westchester, Pennsylvania: Whitford Press.

Gienger, Michael

> 2004   Crystal Power, Crystal Healing. London, U.K.: Blandford

Hay, Louise L.

> 1988   Heal Your Body. Carlsbad, California: Hay House, Incorporated.

Pendulums

Graves, Tom

> 1989   The Elements of Pendulum Dowsing. Shaftesbury, Dorset: Element Books.

Lubek, Walter

> 1998   Pendulum Healing Handbook. Twin Lakes, Wisconsin: Lotus Light
>
> Publications.

Religion

The Bible – several versions available.

Baigent, Michael; Leigh, Richard and Lincoln, Henry

>2005   Holy Blood, Holy Grail Illustrated Edition: The Secret History of Jesus, the Shocking Legacy of the Grail. Delacorte Press.

Brown, Dan

>2003   The Da Vinci Code. New York, New York: Doubleday

Gardner, Laurence

>2002   Blood Line of the Holy Grail: The Hidden Legacy of Jesus Revealed. Fair Winds Press.

Symbols

Chetwynd, Tom

>1982   Dictionary of Symbols. London, Paladin Books: Harper Collins.

Summer Rains, Mary and Greystone, Alex

>1996   Guide to Dream Symbols. Charlottesville, Virginia: Harper Roads Publishing Company.

Reiki

Stein, Diane

>1995   Essential Reiki, A Complete Guide To An Ancient Healing Art. Freedom, CA, The Crossing Press Inc.

Barnett, Libby and Chambers, Maggie

    1996   Reiki Energy Medicine. Rochester Vermont, Healing Arts Press

Foreword by Rand William Lee

    1999   The Original Reiki Handbook of Dr. Mikao Usui. Shangri-La, Lotus Press

Honervogt, Tanmaya

    1998   The Power of Reiki. New York, New York, Henry Holt and Company Inc.

General

Becker, Dr. Robert O. and Gary Selden

    1985   The Body Electric. New York: Quill, William Morrow.

Cameron, Julia

    1992   The Artist's Way. New York, New York: Jeremy P. Tarcher/Putnam.

Davidson, Gustav

    1967   Dictionary of Angels. New York, New York: The Free Press.

Emoto, Masaru

    2004   The Hidden Messages in Water. Hillsboro, Oregon: Beyond Words Publications.

Kroeger, Hanna

> 1973 The Pendulum, The Bible and Your Survival. Hanna Kroeger Publications.

Morgan, Marlo

> 1991 Mutant Message Down Under. New York, New York: Harper Collins.

Redfield, James

> 1993 The Celestine Prophecy. New York, New York: Warner Books Inc.

Walsch, Neale Donald

> 1996 Conversations With God. New York, New York: G.P. Putnam & Sons.

Textbook

> Prescription for Nutritional Healing
> ISBN 7-35918-33077-1

Suggested Internet Resources

There are literally millions of sites on the internet. You may do a "search" to give you a list of sites which contain your key words. It is only by visiting them that you will be able to determine which are useful to you. Don't forget that from one site, you can often be directed to related sites.

What follows is simply a sample of Internet Resources. You are encouraged to extend your search on topics of interest to you.

Aura

http://www.bioenergyfields.org/index.asp?secid=3&subsecid=0

Chakras

https://www.curativesoul.com/Chakras#.XrBe4qhKgdU

https://www.learning-mind.com/7-Chakras-issues/

https://chopra.com/articles/what-is-a-Chakra

https://Chakrasincense.com/

https://diannetrussell.com/energy/articles-2/truth-about-colour/

World Religions

https://www.history.com/topics/religion/bible

http://www.mnsu.edu/emuseum/cultural/religion/

http://www.religion-cults.com/

http://en.wikipedia.org/wiki/Major_world_religions

- Islam
  http://images.google.ca/images?svnum=10&hl=en&lr=&q=islam+symbol&btnG=Search

- Christianity
  http://images.google.ca/images?svnum=10&hl=en&lr=&q=christianity+symbol&btnG=Search

- Hinduism
  http://images.google.ca/images?q=Hinduism+symbol&ndsp=20&svnum=10&hl=en&lr=&start=60&sa=N

  http://www.mnsu.edu/emuseum/cultural/religion/hinduism/beliefs.html

- Buddhism
  http://www.mnsu.edu/emuseum/cultural/religion/buddhism/beliefs.html

- Judaism

http://images.google.ca/images?q=judaism+symbols&ndsp=20&svnum=10&hl=en&lr=&start=40&sa=N

- Traditional Chinese

http://images.google.ca/images?q=Tao+symbols&ndsp=20&svnum=10&hl=en&lr=&start=80&sa=N

- Bahai faith

http://images.google.ca/images?svnum=10&hl=en&lr=&q=bahai+faith+symbol&btnG=Search

https://en.wikipedia.org/wiki/Sanskrit

https://www.ancient.eu/Sanskrit/

Ascended Masters

http://www.dci.dk/en/mtrl/saibabaeng.html

http://www.srisathyasai.org.in/Pages/SriSathyaSaiBaba/Introduction.htm

http://www.greatdreams.com/masters/ascended-masters.htm

http://en.wikipedia.org/wiki/Ascended_master#Examples_of_ascended_masters

http://www.theascendedmasters.com/

http://en.wikipedia.org/wiki/Count_of_St_Germain

Kirlian Photography

http://images.google.ca/images?svnum=10&hl=en&lr=&q=kirlian+photography&btnG=Search

<u>Misc. Info</u>

http://www.zeitgeistmovie.com/Zietgeist

https://www.goodreads.com/book/similar/130686-the-holy-blood-and-the-holy-grail

Tuning Forks

www.Luminati.com

www.somaenergetics.com

https://www.allbodycare.com/tuning-fork-therapy-sound-healing/

https://medium.com/meducated-org/how-to-heal-your-body-by-using-the-frequency-of-life-9307af550fbb

Suggested Video Resources

The film industry has released many movies which depict metaphysical beliefs and phenomena; just a few of them are listed here. While they are fantasy, they may improve your understanding of topics addressed in this course.

1999   What Dreams May Come
   Directed by Vincent Ward

1999   The Sixth Sense
   Directed by M. Night Shayamalan

1999   The Matrix
   Directed by Andy Wachowski and Larry Wachowski

1999   Ninth Gate
   Directed by Roman Polanski

1999   Patch Adams
   Directed by Tom Shadyac

1996   Michael

   Directed by Nora Ephron

1996   Phenomenon

   Directed by John Turtletaub

1991   Stigmata

   Directed by Rupert Wainright

1990   Ghost

   Directed by Jerry Zucker

Message From The Author

To this day, Reiki still mystifies me. I am in awe every day of the power of this life-force energy. Powerful, yet so gentle!

The old saying, 'Wonders never cease to amaze me,' *meaning an expression of surprise used when something unusual or unexpected happens,* really is appropriate for this modality. You will never tire of the miracles you will witness.

Shift happens... Create magic!

Constance

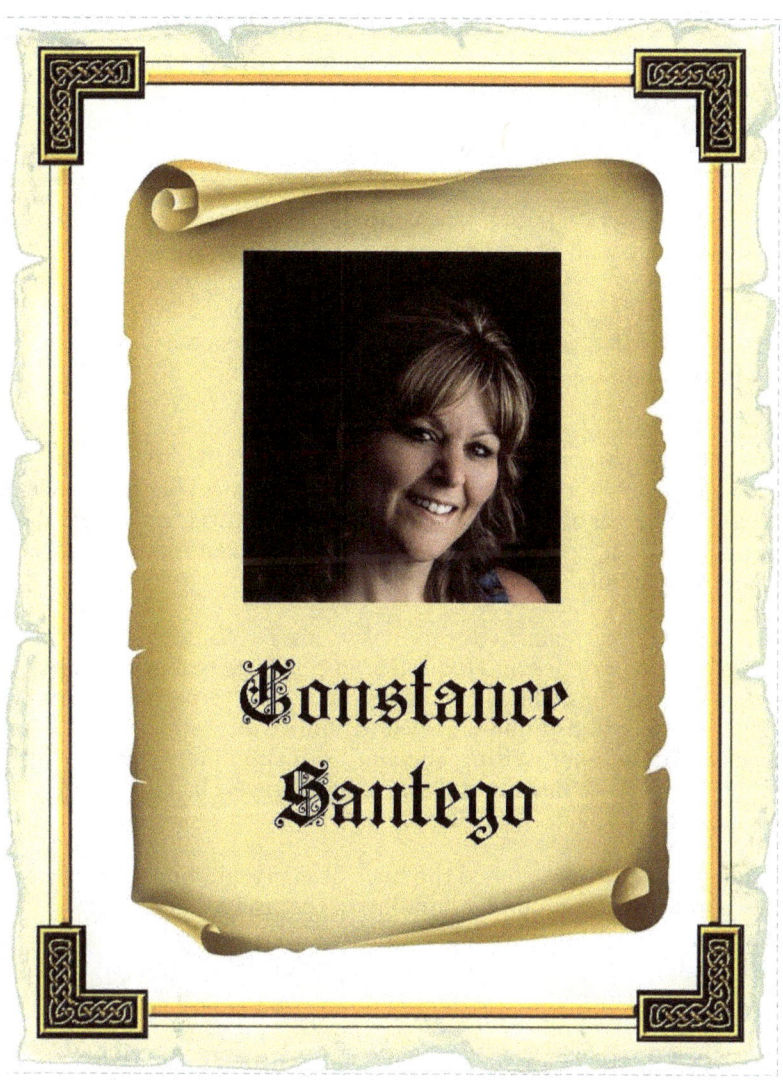

Dream BIGGER!

Dr. Constance Santego is a highly respected expert in the field of holistic health and spiritual healing. With over twenty years of experience teaching courses on these subjects, she has developed a deep understanding of the interconnectedness of the mind, body, and spirit in achieving overall well-being.

Dr. Santego holds a Ph.D. and Doctorate in Natural Medicine, which has provided her with a comprehensive understanding of alternative healing modalities and their application in promoting optimal health. Her educational background has equipped her with the knowledge to address health concerns from a holistic perspective, considering the physical, emotional, and spiritual aspects of an individual's well-being.

Throughout her career, Dr. Santego has been committed to sharing her knowledge and empowering others to take control of their health and healing. She has a unique ability to blend scientific research and traditional wisdom, creating a bridge between conventional and alternative medicine.

In her "Secrets of a Healer" educational series, Dr. Santego draws upon her vast experience and expertise to captivate readers with her insights and teachings. She takes readers on a transformative journey, delving into the realms of holistic health, spirituality, and self-discovery. Through her writing, she aims to inspire individuals to tap into their own innate healing abilities and embrace a balanced and harmonious approach to well-being.

Dr. Santego's work has touched the lives of many, guiding them toward a more profound understanding of themselves and their connection to the world around them. Her series serves as a beacon of wisdom, offering practical tools and techniques for personal growth and transformation.

Overall, Dr. Constance Santego's blend of knowledge, experience, and passion makes her a captivating figure in the field of holistic health and spiritual healing. Her contributions through teaching, writing, and her spellbinding series continue to inspire and empower individuals on their journeys toward well-being and self-discovery.

ALSO AVAILABLE

Play the game *Ikona* – Discover Your Inner Genie

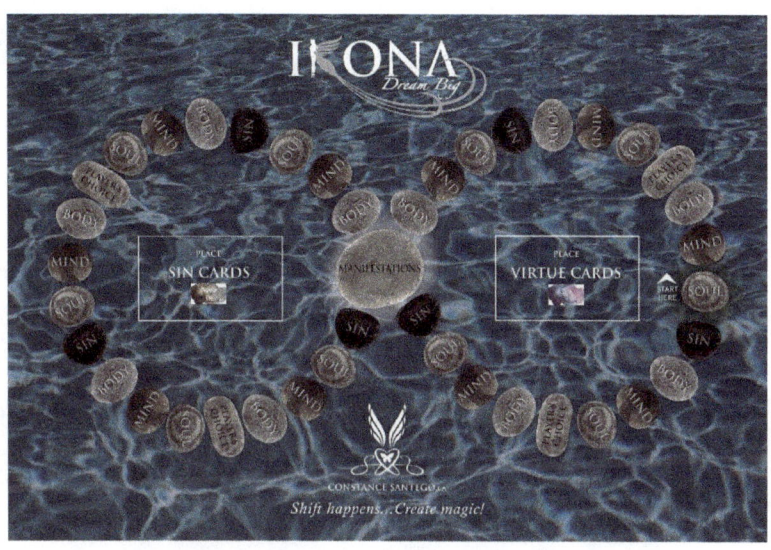

For additional information on

Constance Santego's

wide range of Motivational Products, Coaching Sessions,
Spiritual Retreats,
Live Events and Educational Programs

Go to

www.ConstanceSantego.ca

Follow on Instagram - Constance_Santego and
Facebook - constancesantegoo

Subscribe and receive Free Information and Meditations
on my
YouTube Channel - Constance Santego

www.ingramcontent.com/pod-product-compliance
Lightning Source LLC
Chambersburg PA
CBHW060334030426
42336CB00011B/1335